Age in Place or Find a New Space

How to create beautiful spaces that promote meaningful interactions

Carol Chiang, OTR/L, CAPS, ECHM, CHAMP

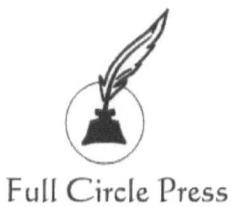

Full Circle Press

© 2025 by Carol Chiang
Published by Full Circle Press, Jacksonville, FL 32256
First Edition, 2025
First Printing

All rights reserved. No part of this publication may be reproduced or transmitted in any form or by any means, electronic or mechanical, including photocopying, recording, scanning or otherwise, or through any information browsing, storage or retrieval system, without permission in writing from the publisher. For more information, contact Full Circle Press, 9564 Glenn Abbey Way, Jacksonville, FL 32256-6491.

Published 2025

10 9 8 7 6 5 4 3 2 1

ISBN-13: 979-8-9910436-0-1 (hardcover)
ISBN-13: 979-8-9910436-3-2 (paperback)
ISBN-13: 979-8-9910436-2-5 (e-book)

Library of Congress Control Number: 2025914226

Age in Place or Find a New Space® is a trademark registered to Carol Chiang. It may not be used in any form without the express permission of the owner.

Evolving Homes® is a trademark registered to Carol Chiang. It may not be used in any form without the express permission of the owner.

DISCLAIMER

Although this publication is designed to provide accurate information in regard to the subject matter covered, the publisher and the author assume no responsibility for errors, inaccuracies, omissions, or any other inconsistencies herein. Further, this publication is meant as a source of valuable information for the reader; however, it is not meant as a replacement for direct expert assistance. If such a level of assistance is required, the services of a competent professional should be sought. The publisher and the author disclaim any and all liability for any claims or injuries that you may believe arose from the following recommendations set forth in this book.

Unless otherwise indicated, all the characters in this book are fictitious. Any resemblance to actual persons, living or dead, is purely coincidental.

Praise for
Age in Place or Find a New Space

Carol Chiang is just absolutely amazing! She's a skilled occupational therapist, a lifelong learner and innovator, and a wonderful mother, friend, and colleague. Her legacy of lending a hand to those who need help improving their functional independence will continue to go on for many generations.

Kenneth Ngo, MD, FAAPM&R
Medical Director, Brooks Rehabilitation Hospital
Medical Director, Brooks Center for Innovation

"Society has missed the mark on how to prepare for the challenges of aging. Planning should be preemptive instead of waiting until an aging mishap occurs. Carol Chiang shares all her years of experience and is masterful in her discussion of how to prepare to age in place. Thank you, Carol, for the good you are putting into the world with this book."

Carolyn McClanahan, M.D., CFP®
Founder, Life Planning Partners, Inc.

"Somehow, Carol approaches the topic of 'aging' with a rare blend of honesty and wisdom that invites us to let go of our fears and biases and instead step into the beauty that can exist in the process of growing older. Whether you're a professional or simply finding yourself walking this path, there's something here that will resonate and offer guidance."

Dawn Heiderscheidt, MOT
CEO & Founder, Aurora Independence

"Carol Chiang's book *Age in Place or Find a New Space* shatters stereotypes about aging and independence by revealing that older adults are not destined for isolation or helplessness but can make empowered choices that fit their unique needs and lifestyles. It is an essential guide for anyone navigating the complexities of aging and housing decisions. Chiang is a giver: with her expertise as an occupational therapist, she provides practical, compassionate advice that empowers readers to plan ahead, whether they wish to modify their current home or explore new living options. Her book is filled with actionable strategies and real-world insights that help individuals and families make confident, informed choices for a safer, more secure, and happier future as they age in place with grace."

Patti Brennan CFP®
CEO Key Financial, Inc.

"Carol succeeds where others have fallen short. She thinks out of the box and grinds until she finds answers to problems that others say are unsolvable. I have seen it time and again. She has earned my trust and highest recommendation."

Dr. David Belkin
Neurofeedback Associates

"I struggle to recall working a shift without at least one patient needing an evaluation for fall-related injuries. This practical, comprehensive guide can help individuals and families prepare before the first fall or re-evaluate a living space after a fall or major hospitalization. I plan to share these tips and recommend this book to my patients, friends, and family."

Kathleen Dumitru, MD
Emergency Physician

"Carol is one of the best clinicians I have ever worked with. Not only do her patients love her, but as a colleague, she is a pleasure to work with. Her skill set is top-notch. She is beyond book smart, and her critical thinking skills always amaze me. When we worked together on a case, I always felt confident that the patient would be in good hands."

Michelle Rosenbaum
Physical Therapist

"Watching my mom's journey from '(almost) perfectly capable' to 'needing a little help' has been an eye-opener for me. Carol's insights are right on point for what we have experienced. Her recommendations for how to gracefully age in place, especially her guidance on taking it one step at a time, have been a source of reassurance for us.

Kim C.
Daughter and Caregiver

"Carol's approach to aging is both forward-thinking and deeply compassionate. She thoughtfully balances physical needs with emotional well-being, empowering individuals to preserve what matters most—both the tangible and intangible—while ensuring they can live safely and independently. Her work is a powerful reminder that it's never too early to start planning."

**Stephanie Miller, Sr. Advisor Marketing
Hartford Funds**

As a coach for healthspan and wellspan, part of my work is helping clients navigate life transitions. This book does a remarkable job of capturing that combination of strategic action and mindset required by both caregivers and those they care for. Yes, your habits in your 20s will absolutely impact your life at age 65, so it's almost never too early or too late to make use of "Age in Place or Find a New Space."

**Ellen Khalifa,
Health Span Habits Coach and Bone Health Peer Educator**

"A visionary blend of occupational therapy, aging, and technology, this book offers a powerful lens into the future of aging well. With clarity and heart, it reframes aging as something to embrace and prepare for, not avoid. It is a testament to the leadership, insight, and innovation that makes Carol one of the best in the field."

**Sydney Marshman, OTD, CEO
Happy at Home Consulting**

"Carol impressed me with her line of questioning. She wanted big picture, rather than focusing on specific areas of pain. She learned where the pain was stemming from based upon my daily routine, habits that included phone usage, driving, sleep habits and posture."

**Jennifer G.
Private Practice Client**

"Aging in place is about living and participating in home and community—doing everything from necessary daily tasks like brushing your teeth to joyous traditions and celebrations such as hosting a holiday celebration. Occupational therapy practitioners are experts in using technology and environmental modifications to keep adults independent and safe in their homes…and Carol Chiang is one of the best!"

**Pamela E. Toto, PhD, OTR/L, BCG, FAOTA, FGSA
Director of the Healthy Home Laboratory, University of Pittsburgh**

"Carol's deep expertise and knowledge makes a profound impact on her clients and the profession of occupational therapy. She dares to push others to innovate and to learn to create a space of independence and a life of purpose. This is a MUST read, to truly understand the art of planning to age successfully in place."

Samantha Lombardi
OTR/L, MBA

"Age in Place or Find a New Space® is an invaluable resource, guiding us through the evolving landscape of technology in aging and making every innovation approachable. By highlighting real-world solutions, it empowers clinicians, care partners, and individuals as they age to create environments that foster dignity, purpose, and connection at every stage of life. Carol's insights remind us that, when thoughtfully integrated, technology becomes not only a universal tool but a compassionate partner in supporting independence and connection for people of all ages."

V Nguyễn, OTD, OTR/L
Tech for Good Innovator & Advocate

"Carol's holistic approach to aging in place goes beyond viewing the built environment as the sole predictor of successful aging. By integrating her occupational therapy expertise with knowledge of universal design, she identifies the full range of factors influencing an individual's desire and ability to remain in their home and community. She also outlines the foundational steps for aging in place and uses examples to highlight the biopsychosocial factors—physical, mental, and social—that support longevity and independence."

**Laura M. Caron-Parker
OT, CAPS, ECHM, FNAP**

"As a fellow OT in the aging-in-place space, this book literally has everything! It's a comprehensive and holistic look at what you need to know to age in the place that you choose. Whether you're concerned about your future or a loved one, this handbook will guide you through the process from every angle."

**Brandy Archie, OTD, OTR/L, CLIPP
Founder, CEO at AskSAMIE.com**

"My wife was about to be released from the hospital within three days, and I felt overwhelmed. Carol's exceptional knowledge allowed me to make my home more accessible to give my wife the spirit of being able to function independently."

L.W.
Husband and Caregiver

"Carol Chiang is brilliant at helping others determine beautiful, tasteful, and affordable solutions to making one's home safe and accessible. Her whole philosophy of empowering people to know what they can do, and "positive aging" is so refreshing."

Snowden McFall
International Speaker

"Carol is truly a special person. Her motivation to change lives is very inspiring. She wholeheartedly advocates for families and the community. It's very apparent that she sees the world differently and is able to solve complex problems with cost-conscious, efficient, and effective solutions."

Dr. Reina Olivera
Doctor of Occupational Therapy

"When we compared the costs of the modifications to the long-term costs of assisted living, it was a 'no brainer' to make the necessary changes and allow our mom to age in place."

Sandy J.
Daughter and Caregiver

This book is dedicated to the millions of caregivers globally.

May equal access to knowledge result in more lightness, laughter, and smiles for you and your families.

"There are only four kinds of people in the world: those who have been caregivers, those who are currently caregivers, those who will be caregivers and those who will need caregivers."
— *Rosalyn Carter*

To my Jackpot girls, you are my rocks.

To my family, you believed in me, and I am eternally grateful.
I love you all so much.

Table of Contents

FOREWORD XIX
PREFACE XXIV
CHAPTER ONE 1
YOUR FUTURE STARTS NOW 1
    Mobility Needs Aren't Just Retirement Needs 2
    Aging in Place Starts in Your 20s 3
    Your Habits Shape Your Options 3
    What You Do Now Determines What You'll Be Able to Do Later 5
    Sitting Is the New Smoking 5
    Final Thoughts: Aging Is Not a Disease 6
    Key Takeaways 7

CHAPTER TWO 8
THE TRUE COST OF AGING IN PLACE 8
    When to Plan Remodels 10
    Many Chances to Get It Just Right 11
    The Shocking Cost of Care 12
    How Much Should I Save? 15
    Who is Best Suited to Aging in Place? 17
    Preparing Your "Age in Place or Find a New Space®" Plan 17
    Be Prepared, Not Panicked 20
    Have a Plan Long Before You Retire 21
    Final Thoughts 21
    Key Takeaways 22

CHAPTER THREE 23
PRACTICAL CHALLENGES OF AGING IN PLACE 23
    The Person-Environment-Occupation Model 25
    How the PEO Model Changes as You Change 26
    Aging in Place Skills 27
    The Evolving Homes® Model 29
    What This Looks Like in Real Life 30
    Final Thoughts 30
    Key Takeaways 31

CHAPTER FOUR 32
WHAT IS UNIVERSAL DESIGN? 32
    Universal Design Principles 32
    Future-Proofing Your Home: Designing with Everyone in Mind 34

VISITABILITY: BECAUSE EVERYONE DESERVES A WAY IN	36
ADA VS. UNIVERSAL DESIGN: WHY ADA RULES DON'T FIT YOUR HOUSE	36
FINAL THOUGHTS	37
KEY TAKEAWAYS	39

CHAPTER FIVE 40
WHY PEOPLE RESIST—AND HOW TO GENTLY SHIFT THE MINDSET 40

DENIAL OF PHYSICAL CHANGES	41
FEAR OF LOSS	41
AVOIDANCE OF THE ISSUES	43
TOO MANY DECISIONS	44
LONGTIME HOMEOWNERS	45
NOT ENOUGH MONEY	46
TRY BEFORE YOU BUY	47
SUCTION GRAB BARS ARE A GATEWAY DRUG	49
GRAB BAR STIGMA	51
LIKE SEATBELTS IN A CAR	52
DO IT FOR THE GRANDCHILDREN	52
UNAWARE OF BEAUTIFUL OPTIONS	53
IMPROVE RESALE VALUE	54
USE OBJECTIVE DATA TO START A CONVERSATION	55
YOU'LL BE IN THEIR SHOES SOMEDAY: REFRAMING THE CONVERSATION	56
THE ANSWER IS SOMEWHERE IN THE MIDDLE	56
SIX INCHES IS STILL PROGRESS: THE POWER OF TINY WINS	57
FINAL THOUGHTS	58
KEY TAKEAWAYS	59

CHAPTER SIX 60
HOME MODIFICATION 60

EXTERIOR ACCESSIBILITY	61
FRONT DOOR	64
GARAGE	68
LAUNDRY ROOM	71
HALLWAY	73
THE STORY BEHIND REASSURANCE RAILS	76
WHEN SAFETY LOOKS LIKE DESIGN	76
LIVING ROOM	78
FURNITURE SELECTION	80
KITCHEN	85
FLEXIBLE AND ACCESSIBLE KITCHEN SOLUTIONS	88
HOME OFFICE	89
FLOORING MATTERS: THE MEMORY FOAM MISTAKE	92
GUEST BEDROOM/EXERCISE ROOM	93
DESIGNING AN EXERCISE SPACE	96
GUEST BATHROOM	97

    BLOCKING: THE UNSUNG HERO OF HOME PLANNING 100
    WHY RETROFITTING IS RISKY 101
    MASTER BEDROOM 102
    BED MOBILITY: GETTING IN, GETTING OUT, AND MOVING WITH CONTROL 105
    MASTER CLOSET 107
    FUTURE-PROOFING: BUILDING WITH TOMORROW IN MIND 109
    MASTER BATHROOM 110
    OT-DESIGNED HOME ASSESSMENT PLATFORMS 121
    NO-CONSTRUCTION SOLUTIONS: ADAPTING WITHOUT REMODELING 115
    LUXURY ACCESSIBILITY: WHY BEAUTY AND FUNCTION MUST COEXIST 116
    THE EVOLVING HOMES® LUXURY ACCESSIBILITY TUB-TO-SHOWER CONVERSION 117
    THE PSYCHOLOGY OF CALM 119
    BIOPHILIC DESIGN: NATURE AS THERAPY 120
    FINAL THOUGHTS: YOUR SPACES THROUGH THE EYES OF AN OT 122
    KEY TAKEAWAYS 123

CHAPTER SEVEN 124

PHYSICAL FITNESS 124

    FALLS ARE AN EPIDEMIC 125
    THE VICIOUS CYCLE OF FALLS 125
    THE ORIGIN OF EVOLVING HOMES® 127
    THE CYCLE OF DECLINE 129
    THE CYCLE OF MISINFORMATION 131
    PROTECT THE LIFE YOU LOVE 133
    PHYSICAL FITNESS IS BRAIN FITNESS 134
    PHYSICAL FITNESS IS LIKE MONEY IN THE BANK 135
    PHYSICAL FITNESS RESTORES SYMMETRY AND BALANCE 135
    PHYSICAL FITNESS BREAKS THE PAIN CYCLE 136
    PHYSICAL FITNESS CAN INSPIRE YOU TO BE YOUR BEST SELF 137
    START SMALL. START TODAY. JUST START. 137
    FIND WHAT MOVES YOU 139
    EASY EXERCISES TO DO IN FRONT OF THE TV 140
    COMBINING EXERCISE WITH FUN 142
    HOW TO DITCH THE CYCLE OF VICIOUS FALLS 144
    FINAL THOUGHTS 145
    KEY TAKEAWAYS 146

CHAPTER EIGHT 147

LIFESTYLE MEDICINE 147

    WHY LIFESTYLE MEDICINE MATTERS 148
    OBSTACLES AND MINDSET SHIFTS 149
    YOUR HABITS ARE YOUR MEDICINE 150
    THE POWER OF ROUTINES 151
    BUILDING MICRO-HABITS 151
    TECH THAT HELPS YOU SUCCEED 152

URINARY TRACT INFECTIONS: A HIDDEN THREAT TO AGING IN PLACE 154
FOOD IS MEDICINE: BUILDING CALM FROM THE INSIDE OUT 155
FINAL THOUGHTS: YOU ARE THE ARCHITECT OF YOUR LIFE 156
KEY TAKEAWAYS.. 157

CHAPTER NINE 158
TECHNOLOGY IN THE HOME 158

SMART HOME TECHNOLOGIES FOR AGING IN PLACE.. 159
PRIVACY CONCERNS WITH SMART HOME TECHNOLOGY 167
NON-WI-FI OPTIONS.. 168
HOW TO GET STARTED... 169
HOW TO LEARN MORE ABOUT ALEXA 169
WHERE TO LEARN MORE ABOUT DIGITAL LITERACY 171
HELPFUL RESOURCES TO PROTECT YOURSELF FROM SCAMS 173
FALL DETECTION TECHNOLOGY 174
TECH SOLUTIONS TO SOLVE TRANSPORTATION CHALLENGES 183
HOME SUPPORT SERVICES THAT LIGHTEN THE LOAD 185
MEDICATION DELIVERY: SIMPLIFY YOUR ROUTINE... 187
SPACE-SAVING FURNITURE: AUTOMATED MURPHY BEDS.................................... 187
MEDICAL CARE WELLNESS SPACES 187
DIAGNOSIS VIA VOICE 189
HIGH-TECH TOILETING 190
CHALLENGES AND SOLUTIONS FOR RURAL POPULATIONS GLOBALLY 190
INTERSECTION OF HEALTHCARE + ROBOTICS 196
MO-GO AND ARTERYXX: SMARTER MOBILITY THROUGH COLLABORATION 198
FUTURE APPLICATION OF ROBOTICS.. 197
FROM MILITARY MISSIONS TO EVERYDAY SOLUTIONS 199
TECHNOLOGY GIVES INDEPENDENCE 201
FINAL THOUGHTS: THE FUTURE OF THE HOME AS A CARE PARTNER 202
KEY TAKEAWAYS.. 203

CHAPTER TEN 204
CAREGIVING RELATIONSHIPS 204

CAREGIVERS ARE SUPERHEROES.. 204
WHY CAREGIVERS MATTER 207
THE EMOTIONAL SIDE OF CAREGIVING.. 208
YOU HAVE AN ARMY: AARP'S TOOLBOX FOR CAREGIVERS.................................. 209
AARP HOMEFIT GUIDE & HOMEFIT APP 210
TIPS TO PROTECT YOUR BODY AND SANITY 210
HOW TO STAY CONNECTED 212
HOW TO PRESERVE MODESTY AND DIGNITY 212
FINAL THOUGHTS: YOU ARE NOT ALONE IN THIS JOURNEY................................. 214
KEY TAKEAWAYS.. 215

CHAPTER ELEVEN 216

AGE IN PLACE OR FIND A NEW SPACE® 216
    MAKE DECISIONS BASED ON YOUR VALUES 218
    WHAT TO LOOK FOR AT AN OPEN HOUSE: THROUGH OT EYES 219
    CASE STUDY #1: WE'RE NOT LEAVING OUR NEIGHBORHOOD! 221
    CASE STUDY #2: DO THE HOMEWORK, FIND THE PEACE 221
    CASE STUDY #3: DOWNSIZING ISN'T FOR EVERYONE 223
    CASE STUDY #4: WHEN IT'S TIME TO PIVOT 226
    FINAL THOUGHTS 228
    KEY TAKEAWAYS 229

CHAPTER TWELVE 230

AGING IN PLACE WITH PARKINSON'S DISEASE 230
    MY JOURNEY WITH PARKINSON'S DISEASE 231
    UNDERSTANDING PARKINSON'S DISEASE 234
    MEDICATION VS. MOVEMENT: WHY EXERCISE IS MEDICINE 235
    BEYOND GENERAL EXERCISE: WHY PARKINSON'S-SPECIFIC MOVEMENT MATTERS 235
    ENVIRONMENTAL STRATEGIES FOR PARKINSON'S SAFETY AND INDEPENDENCE 238
    PARKINSON'S-SPECIFIC PRODUCT IDEAS 243
    MOVING WATER CAN'T FREEZE 246
    FIND YOUR TRIBE 248
    FINAL THOUGHTS 248
    KEY TAKEAWAYS 250

CHAPTER THIRTEEN 251

EPILOGUE 251
    THE FOUR CORNERSTONES OF THRIVING AT HOME 253
    PREPARING, NOT JUST PLANNING 254
    CAREGIVING: THE HEART OF AGING IN PLACE 255
    THE GLOBAL AGING SHIFT: AN INVITATION TO INNOVATE 255
    HEALTHY HABITS ARE FREE 256
    FINAL THOUGHTS: YOUR NEXT STEP STARTS TODAY 256

ONE LAST THING. 257

HOW I PRACTICE WHAT I PREACH: STAYING READY FOR THE NEXT ADVENTURE 257

APPENDIX A: TOOLS & RESOURCES 260
    AGE IN PLACE OR FIND A NEW SPACE®: PLANNING TOOL 267
    ALTERNATIVE LIVING OPTIONS 269
    QUESTIONS TO ASK AFTER A FALL 272

APPENDIX B: FINANCIAL HELP RESOURCES 277
    IS THERE FINANCIAL HELP FOR HOME MODIFICATIONS? 277

APPENDIX C: CLINICIAN RESOURCES 279

PEO MODEL: HOW DO THEY WORK TOGETHER? 279
HOW EVOLVING HOMES® AGING IN PLACE MODEL CONNECTS TO THE PEO MODEL 280
HOW TO USE THE PEO MODEL TO IDENTIFY SOLUTIONS 280
AFTER A FALL: #OT BRAIN INVESTIGATION QUESTIONS 283

APPENDIX D: RESOURCES 286

PRACTICAL CARE & DAILY SUPPORT 290
MEDICAL & HEALTH CONDITIONS 291
FINANCIAL & LEGAL GUIDANCE 292
EMOTIONAL WELLNESS & RESPITE 293
TECHNOLOGY & TOOLS 294
HOME MODIFICATION & AGING IN PLACE 295
HOME ASSESSMENT PLATFORMS 296
FINDING A HOME MODIFICATION OCCUPATIONAL THERAPIST 297
INTERNATIONAL RESOURCES 298
FINDING A CONTRACTOR FOR HOME MODIFICATIONS 299
FINDING DURABLE MEDICAL EQUIPMENT 302
HEALTHY HABITS & FITNESS PROGRAMS FOR AGING ADULTS 305
FINANCIAL ASSISTANCE FOR CAREGIVING 308
EMOTIONAL SUPPORT, SELF-CARE & SUPPORT GROUPS FOR CAREGIVERS 311
DRIVING ASSESSMENT & TRANSPORTATION ALTERNATIVES FOR OLDER ADULTS 314
DIGITAL LITERACY FOR OLDER ADULTS & CAREGIVERS 317
PROTECTING SENIORS FROM ONLINE SCAMS & FINANCIAL EXPLOITATION 320
DISEASE-SPECIFIC FOUNDATIONS & SUPPORT ORGANIZATIONS 323

ACKNOWLEDGEMENTS 329

ABOUT THE AUTHOR 332

Foreword

When Carol approached me to write the foreword for her book, a capture of her life's thought working as an occupational therapist (OT), I had to ask her twice: "Why do you want a designer like me to write the foreword for an OT's book?"

It was a real question for me, but some thoughts shortly followed as we talked about it. Our role titles may differ, as I am a designer and she is an OT, but our missions mirror each other. Improving lives, serving humanity, and evolving the old paradigms of care across the age spectrum. All these sit within the engine room of our individual practice. This drives us both, and it always felt like a core belief from the moment we met, to the hours we spent working together to imagine and enable better spaces for people to age in.

I often joke that neither designers nor OTs need to set alarm clocks as the work draws us automatically into the day. It is the empathic call of the heart, enticing us into action. We do not just rearrange furniture, fix grab handles, or modify routines, but we create surroundings that support and that enable, no matter where a person is on the care journey. OTs and designers (especially those working in inclusive design, universal design, or design for all) both reimagine what it means to live fully and with dignity, purpose, and presence for individuals, carers, groups, and the extended family network.

When my father experienced a stroke many years ago, an OT described his sudden disability as a "stone lobbed into a still pond, its ripples affecting all of us around." That analogy prepared us for the reality of what came next and gave us the permission to be affected. Countless numbers of us will have to stand in the sunshine of an OT's shadow when circumstances change and we feel the impact on our loved ones. If you have ever experienced this, you will know that OTs are often the unsung heroes who care us through calamity.

Another reflection also crossed my mind as I wrote these words, fresh from a conversation with Carol. Designers and OTs can walk through walls. Both professions are non-threatening, which means that in the organisational context they often work in, they do not face the limits that certain departments might. This means that we can be the cement between the bricks, holding a care system together and helping imagine better ones for hospital, community and home settings.

Carol and I both live at the crossroads of function and feeling, of strategy and soul. We care not just about outcomes, but about journeys. And we are both passionate about shaping futures that people actually want to live in.

I was honoured when Carol asked me to write this foreword. Not just because I admire her work, which I absolutely do, but because her book goes far beyond the technical and into the human territory that truly matters. I like to describe this as the emotional architecture of ageing. Yes, this can be seen as a book about environments, but importantly, I also see it as a blueprint for empowerment. It reminds us that ageing is not just about urgency and emergency; it also needs contemplative thinking and strategic planning. It requires silence and listening so we can see what is actually needed and then act on it. These pages give us faith as a springboard to impact, not fear firing us into disarray like a badly aimed starter pistol.

Carol's book teaches us that more thoughtful beginnings give us better endings, especially in the critical area of care.

Carol writes like she lives her professional life, building connections and networks with clarity, compassion, and a calmness that comes from courage. She speaks the language of human dignity fluently, something that all of us need in the minutes of our lives. She brings decades of clinical experience, but also the heart of someone who has sat beside pain, held the space for others, and transformed those experiences into innovation.

I am still struck by the story she tells of working with a multinational company whose engineers designed a robot to help pick older people up from the floor if they have had a fall. They designed it to pick them up as a parent would pick up a baby, but Carol educated them on which part of the older adult body actually needs support. For her, this was not an act of recovery, but one of gentle and generous protection.

In this book, she does not just provide advice, but she accompanies the reader, chapter by chapter, like a wise and trusted guide with the cadence and rhythm of a storyteller.

As I went through Age in Place or Find a New Space, I found myself pausing often, not just to analyse, but also to reflect. A good book does this, making you pause, reread, and annotate its ideas as they find a place in your mind. Carol's words reflect back to us the quiet yet potent truths that we should hear yet sometimes avoid: that we are all ageing; that our bodies will change; and that the way we move through space, such as our homes, our lives, our relationships will also change, too. It helps us to come to grips with this on our own terms.

For me, Chapter 10, which focuses on caregivers, resonated deeply as someone who fulfils that role myself. Carol's humanity shines bright, patterning thoughtfulness into the pages. Her expertise is born from her experience, blending information with inspiration. She honours the caregiver as both everyday hero and silent sufferer, reminding us that behind every ageing parent, spouse, or sibling is someone bending under invisible weight, loving without limits, and often without rest. This continues to resonate, in both my inner world and in the external world I see around me.

As someone who has led conversations about empathy and design across continents, I felt deeply moved by this chapter. Because caregiving, at its core, is creative leadership in its purest form. It demands empathy in connecting, clarity in thought, and creativity in addressing everyday situations. It is the ability to see and serve another person's needs whilst balancing them with your own. It is the courage to keep showing up again and again. These are the same traits I teach aspiring leaders across the world. My own book starts with these words:

This is a story for three types of people. Established leaders, emerging leaders, and the biggest group of all. Those who were never built to be leaders. I sit firmly in that last group.

So, when I look at the work of OT quietly enacted in bedrooms, bathrooms, and kitchens by people with no titles and no applause, I realise that these words are also for them. OTs, like designers, are leaders already. We just need to see them and celebrate them.

And going back to the caregivers who are the focus of Chapter 10, well, Carol gives them voice, structure, and validation as well as tools that are practical, beautiful, and even life-affirming.

As someone who believes in the power of environments to shape identity, I found Carol's approach to inclusive design (my professional focus for the last quarter of a century) to be refreshing and revelatory. Her recommendations are not just about safety or legislation but also about aspiration and delight. They make the inarguable case for everyone's right to live on their own terms, surrounded by beauty, meaning, and grab bars that do not look like they escaped the nearest medical institution!

Carol has the rare ability to speak to both the head and the heart. She knows the codes, the stats, and the guidelines, but she never loses sight of the person behind them, who they are actually created for. To read this book is to awaken parts of ourselves that want to age consciously, one of the warmest gifts that we can give to our future selves, our families, and our potential caregivers.

So, back to the question: Why should a designer write a foreword for an OT's book? Because in a world of increasing complexity, our silos must crumble and disciplines need to speak to each other and more importantly listen to each other. Because the future of care, design, health, and humanity depends on wisdom born from interdisciplinary conversations. Because the best solutions are rarely found in isolation but come from collaboration. Because ageing should not be seen as just a medical issue, but as a social one, deeply ingrained in the human experience across millennia.

I think that this book might just be one of the most important chapters in that story. So, to Carol, thank you for your clarity and courage in writing it, and your call to action that sits in its pages.

And to you, the reader, may this book empower you to age not just in place, but with planned purpose and peace.

Wishing you Joy, Faith, and Grace.

Rama Gheerawo, July 2025
Author of "Creative Leadership: How to Design the 21st Century Organisation."
Penguin Random House
Director and Founder, INSTILL
Creative Leadership | Inclusive Design | Accessibility

Preface

When I was growing up, *MacGyver* was my favorite show. That guy could fix anything with a paperclip, a shoelace, and some duct tape. I was hooked. Not because I wanted to be on TV, but because I loved the idea that no matter how tricky the situation, there was always a way out if you could stay creative and calm under pressure.

Fast forward 30 years, and here I am—a real-life MacGyver. Except, instead of escaping exploding warehouses, I solve problems inside real homes for real people who want to live independently for as long as possible.

As an occupational therapist (OT), I'm a professional problem-solver. I help people live intentionally and with confidence, regardless of age or ability.

As occupational therapists, we're part of a bigger team—joining forces with physical therapists, speech-language pathologists, and others to support people in a holistic way. Together, we look at the full picture: not just how someone moves, but how they live, where they live, and what matters most to them.

Our focus is deeply client-centered. It's not just about restoring function—it's about making sure a person's environment supports the activities that bring them purpose, joy, and meaning.

That's why, when I walk into a client's home, I'm not only assessing for grab bars or measuring bed height. I'm looking at the big picture. I'm watching how they move through their day — how they get out of bed, how they reach for their favorite coffee mug, how they rise from a chair, or carry a basket of laundry without tripping over a rug.

I'm evaluating the lighting, the layout, and the natural flow of movement. I'm identifying risks but more importantly, I'm identifying potential solutions. My job is to make sure the home fits the person, not the other way around.

Planning is a critical part of that process. Ideally, every home remodel should include design features that not only support aging in place but also make the space more inclusive and visitable for guests of all abilities.

Redesigns should consider changing physical needs, such as decreased visual acuity or mobility. Installation of automatic underbed lighting is an easy solution that makes getting to the bathroom in the middle of the night safer and easier to navigate for everyone.

In the bathroom, grab bars are most effective when installed at a height tailored to the homeowner and positioned in a sequence that supports safe movement and proper body mechanics.

In the living room, trip hazards like high-profile rugs and scattered pet toys are relocated to minimize the risk of falls.

In the rest of the home, I clear cluttered walkways to create open and welcoming spaces that feel safe and inviting. These seemingly small details make a big impact, because aging in place isn't just about staying in your home. It's about living safely, comfortably and independently.

Remodels and upgrades, even small ones, come with a cost, and that cost requires planning. Yet most people don't think about these changes when their homes are first built or when they move into a new one. Instead, they often wait until the last minute—right before a knee replacement surgery or after a diagnosis of a neurodegenerative condition—before asking, *"How am I going to safely shower or use the bathroom now?"*

By then, the options are more limited, more expensive, and more stressful. For example, most homes aren't built with the proper wall blocking to securely install grab bars. That means we're left drilling through tile during a crisis, with fingers crossed that the stud finder is accurate ... not an ideal situation when time and safety are on the line.

That's why I believe in planning early and collaboratively. When I work with clients on remodeling projects, I often work with their financial planners to ensure they're prepared, whether it's updating their current home or purchasing one that's easier and more cost-effective to modify.

Planning for the future financially is not what most people expect when they think about occupational therapy but maybe it should be.

After all, when you plan for a growing family, you budget for everything you think the baby will need — the crib, the stroller, and college tuition. Aging in place deserves the same level of foresight and investment, especially if your goal is to remain in your home safely and independently.

In this book, I'll take you beyond the stereotypes of accessibility. You'll see why aging in place starts in your 20s, and I'll help you understand the true cost of aging in place.

We'll explore what healthy habits and routines you can work on now and what things you can do for little to no cost that will pay many dividends later.

This isn't about fear or decline. My hope is that you'll feel empowered to see your home with fresh eyes and a renewed perspective—ultimately inspiring you to take meaningful steps toward creating a beautiful space that evolves with your needs.

Chapter One

Your Future Starts Now

When I talk to friends about my work, one of the things that surprises them most is that I don't just work with older adults. Yes, I'm an occupational therapist (OT) who specializes in aging in place but my work isn't only for people in their 70s and 80s. My clients are often much younger, and here's why.

Mobility issues can happen at any stage of life. Break a leg in your twenties? You've got a mobility challenge. Develop MS in your thirties, arthritis in your forties, or ALS in your fifties? Your mobility, and your independence, is at risk. Parkinson's in your sixties? That's a long road of adjusting ahead. While we expect to slow down as we age, the truth is that changes in how we move, live, and function can happen way before retirement.

As an occupational therapist, I'm always client-focused. I look at you as a person holistically—what issues you're dealing with, look at the environment in which you live, and assess how you're getting around in your environment and how you are completing self-care tasks (what we call your activities of daily living), and I figure out how you could do things more efficiently. Then, I help you decide what you need to do to make your environment fit your specific needs and challenges.

I help you plan your space, not just for now, but for what challenges you may face in the future. I work with interior designers and contractors to shape spaces that truly support you. I work with your financial advisor to help you afford the changes at every stage of life. And I rally your family or support system to keep everyone on the same page.

Mobility Needs Aren't Just Retirement Needs

When you're shopping for your first home, you're probably not thinking about your needs at age 85. But accessibility isn't just for "old age", it's comfort and convenience for *everyone*. Think about it: lever handles are easier when your hands are full of groceries. Wide doorways make moving a stroller or a wheelchair seamless. Zero-step entries reduce tripping hazards and make it easier for kids, pets, and guests to come and go. Buying a home with features like this makes everyone's life easier, including yours if you decide to have children.

Have you ever thought about how tough it can be to navigate stairs with a stroller? My sister used to haul my nephew up four concrete steps every time she came home from the park. It was exhausting, and honestly, it made her less likely to leave the house in the first place. When your environment works against you, it limits your options. It discourages engagement with the outside world, which is essential for our mental and emotional well-being.

What about installing handrails on both sides of the staircase instead of just one? They're just as helpful for a toddler learning to navigate steps as they are for an older adult with poor vision or balance issues. Secure handholds in the bath or shower benefit both young children and grandparents, making those transfers safer and easier. These are small design choices that offer big support for everyone, at every stage of life.

C1 | Your Future Starts Now

Grab bars in the shower? My husband and I aren't anywhere near retirement, but we love ours. They're sturdy, stylish, and offer peace of mind, especially after a long day at the beach. There's something reassuring about having a secure handhold when you're rinsing sand off your feet. And a shower bench? Total game-changer for shaving your legs. These aren't signs of aging. They're signs of smart design. If you wait until you need them to install them, you've already waited too long.

Aging in Place Starts in Your 20s

Most people in their twenties are focused on work, relationships, and (maybe) buying their first home. Planning for aging feels like a lifetime away. But according to the AARP Home and Community Preferences survey, nearly three-quarters of adults over 18 say they want to stay in their homes as they age[i]. That goal doesn't happen by accident. It takes foresight and habits that start *now*.

Your future health is built on what you do today. Exercise, eat well, move with intention, and yes, start thinking about your environment. If something unexpected happens (an injury, an illness), how quickly you bounce back often depends on the lifestyle you've built in advance.

Your Habits Shape Your Options

Proactive choices go a long way in delaying the onset and progression of disease. But let's be honest—imagining ourselves decades down the road isn't easy. Still, we have to try. How mobile we'll be in our later years depends on the choices we make today. Regular exercise and honest self-reflection are the cornerstones of healthy aging.

Ask yourself:
- Am I moving enough to keep my joints from getting stiff?
- Am I building lean muscle and maintaining a healthy weight?
- Am I eating foods that keep my energy and blood sugar stable?

Age in Place or Find a New Space

- Am I taking my medications consistently and on time?

Healthy habits aren't complicated but they do require effort. You can either experience the pain of discipline or the pain of regret. When I work with clients, my goal is to help them understand that this investment in their health is absolutely worth it.

Exercise benefits people of all ages and ability levels. We've all heard it helps fend off heart attacks, and that's because it does. A body in motion trains the heart to beat slower and stronger, which means it needs less oxygen to function. It makes arteries more elastic, helping blood flow more efficiently. And it boosts your levels of "good" HDL cholesterol.[ii]

Physical activity also plays a major role in preventing diabetes. Muscles that are regularly used stay responsive to insulin, the hormone that helps usher blood sugar into cells, so blood sugar stays more stable over time.[iv] Even certain cancers like breast, colon, endometrial, and ovarian show lower rates in people who get four to seven hours of moderate to vigorous exercise each week.[iv]

One of my favorite expressions is: "Motion is lotion." The more you move, the more you nourish your joints and your brain thrives on movement and routine. When we move, our blood vessels pump oxygen throughout the body, including to the brain. That means clearer thinking, more energy, and greater motivation. Personally, I don't exercise to fit into skinny jeans. My motivation is sanity over vanity. That's what gets me out the door every day. Brisk walking is my therapy; the rhythm is meditative, grounding, and helps regulate my mood.

Here's the truth: carrying excess weight increases your risk of developing knee arthritis, which is the number one reason for knee replacements. Sugar crashes lead to daytime drowsiness, which wrecks your sleep at night. Taking blood pressure meds late, then doubling up early, causes swings that can knock you off your feet, literally.

Sugar crashes, poor sleep, blood pressure swings—they're more than just annoying. They're dangerous. But the good news? These risks are largely preventable. With the proper routines in place, you can stay stronger, safer, and independent longer.

What You Do Now Determines What You'll Be Able to Do Later

Physical activity isn't just for heart health. It's one of the best defenses against diabetes, obesity, and certain cancers. It improves your mood, memory, and focus. It slows down cognitive decline and boosts emotional resilience. There are studies showing exercise works just as well as antidepressants for mild to moderate depression.

Studies also show that people are more afraid of a dementia diagnosis than they are of death.[iii] Dementia risk is real but it's not inevitable. The evidence is that physical activity can delay the slide of cognitive decline into dementia, and even once the process has started, exercise can improve certain aspects of thinking. Exercise improves blood flow to the brain, staving off cognitive decline.[iv]

Sitting Is the New Smoking

This isn't just a catchy phrase. More and more research is showing that sitting for too long can be just as harmful to your health as smoking is. Being inactive raises your risk for heart disease, diabetes, and even conditions like stroke or certain cancers. Regular physical activity improves heart and lung function; improves memory, thinking, and problem-solving; minimizes depression; and more.[iv]

Every 30 minutes you spend sitting, you miss an opportunity to keep your muscles awake and your joints flexible. You don't need a gym. Just stand, stretch, and walk around. Get into a rhythm of moving before stiffness sets in. Because when it does, you'll be more prone to falls—and once the cycle of falling starts, it's hard to stop.

For people with Parkinson's or arthritis, regular movement is essential. The chance of a fall is two to three times higher than for someone without a serious mobility challenge. Movement reduces the risk of serious injury, supports brain function, and boosts confidence. For every hour you spend not moving, you're training your body to be sedentary. Over time, inactivity becomes the default, not the exception.

Final Thoughts: Aging Is Not a Disease

Let's end this chapter by pushing back on the idea that aging is bad. It's not. Aging is a season of life. But like every season, it takes preparation.

You start losing muscle around age 35. Half a pound a year, unless you do something about it. You will also start gaining two pounds of fat every year if you maintain your current activity level. That's not a crisis—it's a natural aging process called sarcopenia.

It just means that once people hit their 30s, it's time to start adjusting eating habits and adding strength training to keep muscles strong as time passes. Biology responds to action. You can build strength. You can shift habits. You can change your story. So start now. One decision, one habit, one adjustment at a time. Your future self is counting on it.

Key Takeaways

- Mobility challenges can happen at any age, not just in older adulthood.
- Universal design features—like no-step entries and lever handles—benefit people of all ages and stages.
- Planning for accessibility early makes daily life easier now and future-proofs your home.
- Healthy habits formed in your 20s and 30s directly impact your ability to stay mobile later in life.
- Regular exercise improves not just physical health but mental clarity and emotional well-being.
- Sitting for long periods increases your risk of falls, disease, and mobility decline—movement matters.
- Aging is natural, not negative—and building muscle, eating well, and staying active helps you age well.

Chapter Two

The True Cost of Aging in Place

Imagine waiting until your child is 17 years old to start thinking about how you're going to pay for college. The acceptance letters are coming in, the tuition deposit is due, and at that moment, you sit down to figure out if you can afford college. That would feel *completely insane*, right?

Yet that's *exactly* how most people approach aging in place. Most people think, "I'll deal with it later if it happens." They wait until their joints are bone on bone before they see a doctor. They wait until their spouse is burned out from caregiving before looking at respite options. They wait until they have fallen before agreeing to install grab bars.

Listen, aging is a given, so any proactive planning you do now will pay off in both dollars saved and quality of life preserved. And just like planning for college, it's impossible to know how much to save if you don't know how much it costs to make your home aging-in-place-friendly. Do you know how to determine which bathroom safety products are worth the added expense and which aren't? How can you know which retirement communities are a good match for your interests and

C2 | The True Cost of Aging in Place

personality if you haven't been on a tour or talked to the residents there in advance? Aging in place planning shouldn't be a crisis plan—it should be a life plan.

I define aging in place as a purposeful decision to stay in your own home as you get older. It's the decision that, "This is the home and community I love, and I will do anything necessary to allow me to stay here as I get older." In an ideal world, this means that you have also taken the time to dissect what skills are needed to care for yourself and what skills are needed to care for your home.

You will have already explored what the options are if you start to find that accomplishing these tasks is becoming more difficult. You will have visited multiple retirement communities to understand what the costs are and have a short list of the ones that could be potential back-up plans. You will have identified your support system and know how you will keep the meaningful activities in your life going to not feel isolated. And finally, you will have decided on where the line in the sand is to indicate that it's time for the contingency plan to be deployed because the amount of care needed is now too much to handle in the home environment.

This is the ideal situation.

The reality? Aging in place is often used as a default plan. Why? Because it's easy.

People think, "I'm already living independently in the home I love, so why change anything?" The part that people forget is that they are going to be 20 years or 30 years older, and their needs may be quite different depending on how proactive they have been in establishing healthy lifestyle habits early on.

I've had clients say, "I've worked hard my whole life, and now I just want to sleep in, eat what I want, and watch Netflix all day long." I get it. You have the right to live your life the way you want. But ask yourself, is this the retirement you dreamed about? Because in this plan, all roads lead to weakness, falls, and hospitalizations. Or do you want an elevated quality of life that gives you freedom to move and do whatever you want in your life? You don't need to live like an Olympic athlete, but you do need a plan.

The greatest news is that it's the little things you do that can make a big difference in your quality of life and, perhaps more importantly, in your wallet.

When to Plan Remodels

In my career, I've found that most people believe they should consider making changes to their homes only after they retire or after the first time they have a fall.

That's too late.

The time to start thinking about making those changes is as soon as you buy your first house. Every remodel of the kitchen or bathroom gives you the opportunity to research accessibility options, add universal design features, and implement changes that will make it easier for everyone of all ages to live in your home—be it you and your family or someone else—all without incurring significantly more cost. And in your younger years, you may also have more strength, energy, and motivation to trade your sweat equity for a discount in price.

In my experience, if you're building a home, adding universal design features only adds one percent to the total cost of construction. That's compared to the thousands of dollars it costs to remodel those spaces once the house is completed.

If you're remodeling, aim to install blocking in the walls for future grab bars, widen doorways, create barrier-free entrances, and build in automated lights. These small changes can have big impacts on function and more importantly, decrease the stress for you as the homeowner in the event that any of that is needed.

Modifications like zero-threshold entrances will also make life easier for all who live in your home or who just come to visit. From moms pushing strollers to teens with sprained ankles on crutches to older parents with mobility challenges in wheelchairs, everyone benefits.

C2 | The True Cost of Aging in Place

The wonderful thing about slowly improving the spaces in your home is that the cost and the headaches of construction are spread out over time. You'll also be able to benefit from these changes throughout your lifespan rather than only in the last few decades.

Many Chances to Get It Just Right

Do you have clothes in your closet that you thought you would love but have remained mostly unworn? I know I do. Maybe you were trying something new, but it turned out that wasn't really your style. Or perhaps the clearance price was so compelling, you talked yourself into bringing it home.

Opportunities to make "mistakes" are the gift of starting early. Often, the only way you know if you like something is to experience it yourself. That's why making small changes over time and thinking through each remodel for accessibility will set your house up to be ready for you by the time you get to your retirement age.

By then, you'll have had plenty of time and multiple remodels under your belt to figure out what you need and what you like, especially if you start by asking yourself this question: "If I end up deciding to age in place in this house, what are my options, how much do they cost, and are those options important enough to me to include despite the cost?"

And just so you know, expect your preferences to change with experience. Think: walk-in bathtubs. They seem like a great idea until you realize you hate that you get cold waiting for the water to drain before you can open the door and get out, or that you're bathing sitting upright like in a chair with water only to your chest level. Not exactly a true bath.

It is also worth mentioning that many things are a fraction of the cost to do on the front end rather than waiting to address them at the last minute. Poor preparation often leads to spending the same amount of money on temporary fixes as on higher-quality solutions. Wouldn't you rather have more control and choice in your life? I know that I value the efficient use of money.

Age in Place or Find a New Space

When you're building or buying your first home, it's the perfect time to pause and consider whether there are any universal design or accessibility features you might want to incorporate. Even if you're not facing immediate needs, adding these elements now can help you prepare for the unexpected in the future. Taking the time to slow down, explore your options, and make thoughtful decisions will pay dividends for years to come.

Whether you ultimately decide to include these features or not, the most important step is opening your mind to the possibilities early on. This gives you the opportunity to make intentional choices—deciding whether this first remodel is the right time to move forward or if certain upgrades can wait until a future renovation, perhaps a decade from now, if you're still living in the same home.

Sometimes, that first remodel comes with a tight budget. In those cases, you might choose to install the structural supports (blocking) now and postpone larger investments like a walk-in tub until the next remodel. By approaching home improvements gradually, you can spread out the costs and avoid leaving all the critical changes until after you've had a fall or faced a crisis.

The Shocking Cost of Care

People are often stunned when they realize just how expensive care can be.

A friend of mine, who owns a Comfort Keepers franchise in Florida, shared that 24/7 in-home care can easily run upwards of $240,000 a year. Many retirement communities start around $100,000 annually, and memory care—whether at home or in a specialized facility—can cost significantly more. It's a lot to take in, and for most people, it can feel overwhelming.

According to Genworth's Cost of Long-Term Care study,[v] in 2025, the cost to have someone come into your home just 40 hours a week to help you with regular homemaker services costs $5,517 a month. A

C2 | The True Cost of Aging in Place

home health aide costs $6,068 a month. That's 2025. Fast-forward to 2065, and the costs rise exponentially to $17,996 and $19,795 a month, respectively, given just a three percent annual inflation rate change. (See Box 1).

Genworth Calculations Median Monthly Cost 40-hour Week		
In-Home Care	**2025**	**2065**
Homemaker Services	$5,517.00	$17,996.00
Home Health Aide	$6,068.00	$19,795.00
Community & Assisted Living	**2025**	**2065**
Adult Day Health Care	$2,183.00	$7,122.00
Assisted Living Facility	$5,676.00	$18,515.00
Nursing Home Facility	**2025**	**2065**
Semi-Private Room	$9,197.00	$30,001.00
Private Room	$10,326.00	$33,683.00

Box 1[vi]

Age in Place or Find a New Space

Another common pitfall is underestimating how much care you will need in the future and overestimating the amount of care that's going to be available, whether it's a spouse, your kids, or your close friends. Nobody thinks they will need care. It's much easier to imagine that we will drop dead, perfectly healthy, at the ripe old age of 99.

The reality is that for most people, aging will simply mean that the chores we do today without thinking, like cooking for ourselves, cleaning the house, and basic hygienic practices like showering, dressing, and toileting, all will gradually become harder to do the older we get.

And there are other things you may also need help with eventually: home maintenance, mowing the lawn, grocery shopping, doing laundry—the list goes on. In some cases, we may have no choice but to have assistance for each one of these things.

And that can be hard because many of us are fiercely independent and don't want to accept help from a stranger. "I'll probably be married and have grown children by that time. One of them will help me do all that," you might think. There might be some flaws in this thinking.

Not everyone is cut out to be a caretaker, regardless of the vows we made or the strength of the family ties. Caregiving can be physically and emotionally exhausting. I've had more than a few couples look at each other and realize they'd never actually talked about how they'd handle that dynamic.

It's not a fun conversation, but it's a necessary one. The most important thing to recognize is that no one is good at everything. Your mission, should you choose to accept it, is to understand what is in your skill set and what is not. That honest conversation will allow you to move on to the next step, which is making sure that your financial plan includes paid caregivers at a frequency that will provide enough support and self-care for both you and your spouse.

C2 | The True Cost of Aging in Place

How Much Should I Save?

I can't tell you how many times I've heard, "It's cheaper to stay at home." And sometimes, it is. But not always. The difficulty is that when you are comparing the cost of aging in place at home to a senior living community, the costs are presented to you in an all-inclusive price. With your home, you pay your bills as they come due—generally, month by month or once a year. It can be easy to assume that staying home is less expensive when you see a $6,000 a month fee in the brochure.

However, people forget to factor in the cost of care as well as the cost of meeting your physical, social, and emotional needs: $30 an hour for a caregiver to help you bathe, take you to the doctor, and drive you to church after can add up fast. Bills can easily hit $20,000 a month. Then there are the home repairs, the utility costs, the pest control, and the lawn maintenance. Aging in place isn't a free ride. It's a choice that needs to be made with eyes wide open.

When you're planning to age in place, you have to take a look at your whole life, your lifestyle, your expectations for what it would take to stay where you are, or prepare your future dream home. That cost includes more than just the median annual housing cost (assuming you may still have a mortgage or rent to pay to provide a fair comparison to assisted living). The cost also includes the amount of money it would take to make your home suitable for aging in place (making sure you adjust for the cost of living).

To calculate the variable costs, the best way I've found to make a reasonable comparison is by totaling the yearly costs and dividing by 12 for the average monthly cost to live in your home. And don't forget to consider that some costs, such as a new roof every 25 years or a new HVAC every 8-10 years, aren't as easy to break down into that calculation so building in a buffer is a good idea.

Lastly, remember to account for what it costs to stay physically active, like the cost of a gym membership or a personal trainer, and what it will cost to maintain social connections, like lunch with the girls once a week or taking your grandchildren to the zoo.

Age in Place or Find a New Space

Now, let's talk about some situations where aging in place may *not* be the cheaper option.

Deferred Home Maintenance

If someone hasn't updated their home in 20 to 30 years, chances are the space no longer fits who they are today, let alone who they'll be in the decades to come. To safely age in place, they'll likely need to invest in key updates. That might mean installing a security system, reconfiguring the bathroom for better accessibility, or undertaking a full renovation to remove hazards. And while these changes are essential, the costs can add up quickly.

Caregiver Burnout

If the plan is to save money by expecting a spouse to handle 100 percent of the caregiving responsibilities, it's time to rethink that strategy. Caregiver burnout is real and it's devastating. Just look at the numbers: a Stanford University study found that caregivers have a 63 percent higher mortality rate than non-caregivers. Even more sobering, 40 percent of Alzheimer's caregivers die from stress-related disorders before the person they're caring for. The truth is, no one can work 24/7, 365 days a year, without paying a heavy price—physically, emotionally, or financially.[vii]

Chronic Health Conditions

When it comes to the cost of care, lifestyle habits matter. Individuals with less-than-ideal health habits often require a higher level of care—care that can quickly become too expensive to manage at home. Providing around-the-clock assistance means hiring at least three caregivers per day at roughly $30 an hour, which adds up to $240,000 or more annually. In such cases, the complexity and intensity of care may make a skilled nursing facility a more practical and financially sustainable option.

Who is Best Suited to Aging in Place?

In my experience, the people most likely to age in place successfully are those who've prioritized their health throughout life, maintained strong social connections, and consistently kept their homes well-maintained, clutter-free, and thoughtfully updated to meet their evolving needs. They understand that the smartest way to save money in the long run is to invest in their health, because exercise is cheap, but home modifications and medical treatments are not.

Preparing Your "Age in Place or Find a New Space®" Plan

There's a big difference between planning to age in place and truly preparing for it. Planning means you've decided that staying in your home is the goal, but preparation is where the real work begins. Without taking concrete steps to explore your options, understand the costs, or define a backup plan, even the best intentions can leave you scrambling. When you ignore something on the front end, you end up paying twice as much on the back end. And too often, people find themselves in a crisis, with limited choices and sky-high "hurricane prices" for rushed, mediocre solutions.

The smarter alternative? Proactively identify the range of possibilities that could unfold over your lifetime. When you anticipate and plan for future needs, your future self will feel cared for and supported. Gather the facts, do the research, and think through your options. This kind of preparation allows you to make informed decisions, including which tasks you may eventually want or need to outsource. It's not just about hoping for the best. It's about having a strategy if things don't go as planned.

As we've discussed, taking advantage of every remodel to create a safer, more accessible environment is a foundational step toward successful aging in place. But just as important is taking the time to think

Age in Place or Find a New Space

through what your plan will be if life doesn't go as expected. While none of us can predict the future, walking through potential scenarios with clarity and courage, and seeking the answers you need now, means you'll be ready no matter what comes. Think of it like writing your will: these are future-focused decisions made while you're calm, clear-headed, and not under pressure. It's peace of mind, created by design.

This is your Age in Place or Find a New Space® plan.

So, what goes into this folder of backup plans? Everything we have been talking about. Think through what an aging-friendly bathroom would look like. Think about function and not just design.

If you stayed at home, who would be available to help? What kind of help could they provide? Are they the person you would ask to pick up prescriptions for you, or would they be the person who would be comfortable helping you with a shower? How much help can they provide? Is it only after work? Weekends? Do they have their own family to manage? Who could step in if they are sick? You may not have all the answers right now, but knowing who you can call to get the information you need is the first step toward a solid plan.

What will be the breakpoint of when it's too difficult to manage at home? Incontinence, aggression, and heavy lifting with transfers are the biggest reasons people are unable to be cared for at home. Find out from the Genworth Cost of Care Survey what the national median cost for a private room in a nursing home is and what it will cost in your zip code.

File away your research, your proactive decisions, and your parameters. "If my cost of care exceeds this trigger point, my action plan will be to move into a senior living community, and based on my earlier research, I've decided that these will be my top three choices because they have the best mix of choices and value for me."

Your backup plan is put together in moments when there is no urgent need, so you are calm and able to think clearly. A compelling reason to take this step is that everyone in your life who cares about you will immediately calm down. When your inner circle sees that you have

C2 | The True Cost of Aging in Place

taken the future seriously, done the research to know how much it's going to cost, and have contingency plans if things go south, they can take a breath.

This might also be a good time to talk about what your expectations are of them if you do need help down the road. A potential source of anxiety may be the unspoken question of, "If my mom gets sick, will I have to quit my job to take care of her?" Not everyone was built to be a caregiver, and that's okay. You just need to have a plan for it. They worry about you because they love you and want to know that you will be OK. Once you can show them that you have a plan, people will stop pestering you, and you'll be free to do whatever you want.

I have also had couples use this as a survivorship plan. "When one of us passes away, the plan will be that the surviving spouse will move to one of these communities so they won't be lonely and so they will have the support that they need." No one likes to think about the inevitable, but consider these discussions a gift to your future self and your spouse.

When the time comes, you will have the brain space to just grieve your loss and not feel overwhelmed with anxiety about how you will manage life without your partner. In my opinion, the real value of this exercise is peace of mind for your spouse. As a couple, you will have made those decisions together long before you needed them, and knowing that the other one will be supported and taken care of means your sweetheart will heal over time and continue to live the vibrant life you had together, all because you were brave enough to look at it.

In my experience, the people who truly understand the importance of preparing for the future are often those who have cared for their parents. Having navigated the caregiving journey themselves, they possess firsthand insight into what is genuinely needed. They know the real costs—not just financial, but physical and emotional—and they don't need to imagine where they might face challenges in their own lives. As a result, they tend to be far more proactive and significantly better prepared, both financially and emotionally, for what lies ahead.

Be Prepared, Not Panicked

Aging is inevitable, but suffering doesn't have to be. The cost of not preparing is real, and it's heartbreaking to watch hard-earned retirement savings disappear on avoidable care expenses. With a little foresight and planning, so much of that financial and emotional strain can be avoided.

I've seen firsthand how preparation—or the lack of it—can shape an outcome. It reminds me of when I first moved to Florida and encountered hurricane season, something completely foreign to me. Growing up in northern Manitoba, storm preparation meant keeping a shovel and blankets in your car, not tracking a swirling system on the news for days, wondering if you needed to board up your windows or evacuate.

At first, it felt overwhelming. Where do I go if I need to leave? What do I pack? What if the storm changes direction—am I overreacting?

But year after year, I started doing what seasoned Floridians do: I built a plan. I have bins in my garage packed with essentials—flashlights, batteries, documents, food, and water. Once a year I review them, update the contents, and then forget about them. And I do this every year even though in all the years I've lived in Florida, I've never spent a single night in a shelter.

So, why do I keep doing this? Because I know that if the moment ever comes, I won't be scrambling under pressure. I have a plan, which means I can stay calm while others rush to empty the grocery store shelves.

This is exactly the mindset you need when it comes to aging in place. Aging in place is about doing what you can now, while things are calm, so you don't feel stressed or overwhelmed. Your older, wiser self will applaud you for putting the work in on the front end!

Have a Plan Long Before You Retire

The most important thing I want you to take away from this chapter is that the time to prepare your home for aging in place isn't after retirement—it's *before*. Once you stop working, your financial flexibility narrows. Necessary changes like widening doorways, installing a zero-threshold shower, or adding a main-floor bedroom can quickly shift from "wise investment" to "unrealistic expense."

But when you start early, everything changes. If you're still earning, you have options. You can phase upgrades over time. You can plan, pivot, and yes—splurge a little, if you want to. That luxury tub or smart-home tech doesn't have to be out of reach. If it's worth it to you, it's worth planning for.

Don't wait until a fall or a new diagnosis forces you into making decisions that aren't aligned with your values. By the time these things happen, it's often too late to make thoughtful decisions. Instead of feeling prepared, people feel rushed, overwhelmed, and boxed in by options that don't reflect how they want to live. I want you to have a different experience.

Final Thoughts

The goal here isn't perfection. It's readiness. It's knowing all the upgrades to your home have been completed long before you stop working. It's having clarity to know what you want and knowing you have the support to help you get there. You don't have to take every step today. Just start with the questions. Make sure that your future is something you walk into with confidence, not something that catches you off guard.

Age in Place or Find a New Space

Key Takeaways

- Start planning for aging in place early—don't wait for a crisis.
- Use every remodel to add simple, future-friendly upgrades.
- Small changes now cost less than emergency fixes later.
- Aging in place isn't always cheaper; factor in all care and home costs.
- Build a backup plan with clear options and financial triggers.
- Talk with loved ones about caregiving expectations ahead of time.
- Prepare before retirement, when you still have flexibility and resources.

Chapter Three

Practical Challenges of Aging in Place

So, what is Occupational Therapy anyway? This was a great definition presented at the 2025 Australian Occupational Therapy Association Conference by Gail Whiteford:

"Occupational therapy is a justice-oriented profession. Occupational therapists work alongside people to ensure they are included and can participate in society through doing, being, becoming, and belonging in their communities and living lives characterized by purpose and dignity in ways that are culturally meaningful and sustainable." (Whiteford, 2025)

Occupational therapists help people do the things that matter most to them, especially when life starts to get a little harder. But many people don't realize what our role is or how we differ from physical therapy. It's a common misunderstanding, one I encountered regularly in my own work.

For 13 years, I worked as a Home Health Occupational Therapist. Every Sunday, my job was to schedule OT evaluation visits for all my

Age in Place or Find a New Space

new patients. Given the confusion about what we do, these calls often went something like this:

> **Me**: "Hi, my name is Carol Chiang. I'm an occupational therapist. Your doctor has prescribed OT, and I'm calling to schedule a visit."
>
> **Patient**: "You seem very nice, but I think there's been a mistake. I'm retired. I had a hip replacement last week, so I only need PT to rehab my hip and get back to golfing."
>
> **Me**: "Actually, my role is to help you regain independence with things like dressing, bathing, and grooming, as well as getting in and out of bed or on and off the toilet. I can also offer suggestions for managing household chores while you recover."
>
> **Patient**: "Hmm, that makes sense. The doctor said I can't bend past 90 degrees for three months. That'll make cleaning my cat's litter box tricky. Maybe you should come out."
>
> **Me**: "Absolutely. And while I'm there, I can show you how to use a reacher, sock-aid, and long-handled shoehorn to help with dressing. You wouldn't want to show up on the golf course without pants on, right?"

Occupational therapy is about the job of living. Your "occupation" includes everything that makes up your day: getting dressed, cooking meals, walking the dog, managing medications, or hugging your grandchild without pain. These are the everyday tasks that create a meaningful life, and those are your jobs.

As OTs, we're trained rehab professionals; we are human-centered, so we don't start by telling you what to do. We start our investigation by asking for more information:

C3 | Practical Challenges of Aging in Place

- How do you take care of yourself?
- What parts of your routine are getting harder?
- What's most important to you?
- What brings you joy?
- What would you hate to give up?

From there, we build personalized solutions around your goals and values. We're creative, collaborative problem-solvers. You tell us your non-negotiables, and we figure out the "how." Why? Because if it matters to you, it matters to us.

We also break things down into manageable steps. We meet you where you are and help keep you doing what you love, in the place you love, for as long as possible. #otbrain #professionalproblemsolver

The Person-Environment-Occupation Model

How do OTs know what to look for? We use a framework called the Person–Environment–Occupation (PEO) Model.[viii] It helps us identify where the disconnects are that might be limiting your success and how to fix them.

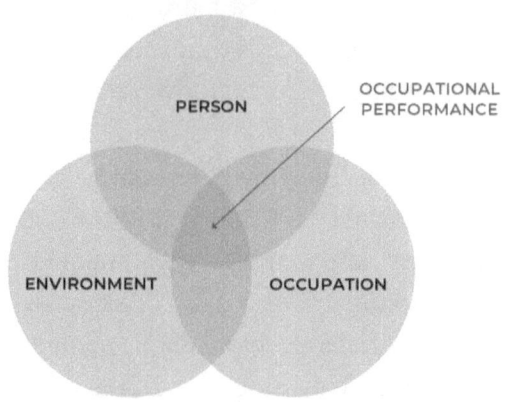

Age in Place or Find a New Space

Here's a breakdown of each domain:

- **Person**: This includes your roles, beliefs, personality, health, cognition, physical skills, and sensory abilities.
- **Environment**: Your physical home, the social or cultural norms of your community or care setting, and even financial access to resources.
- **Occupation**: The tasks and activities that bring meaning and structure to your day, from brushing your teeth to gardening or volunteering.

When these three domains align, your quality-of-life increases; when they don't, performance suffers.

How the PEO Model Changes as You Change

The PEO Model isn't static—it evolves with you. What's the right fit today may not be the right fit tomorrow, and I've experienced that firsthand.

When my husband and I moved to Florida, we lived in the cutest little one-bedroom apartment—600 square feet of manufactured charm, complete with three concrete steps and a "garden" (really just dirt and hope). At the time, it was perfect. No kids. No clutter.

A year later? Same space, but now with two adult bikes stored in the pantry. Cooking became a yoga-meets-obstacle-course experience. My performance didn't decline, my environment did.

So we moved to a 1,100-square-foot townhome. Boom—dinner got easier, and life felt less chaotic. Then we had our first baby. Our neighbor also got a roommate, with a full drum set, whose room shared a wall with the nursery. You can guess what happened next.

We moved again. This time to a 2,500 square foot home. I was nine months pregnant and closed on the house the same week I had a C-section. (Would not recommend.)

C3 | Practical Challenges of Aging in Place

That move worked because the environment finally supported our roles.

Later, in my 40s, I noticed my body changing—muscle loss from aging and perimenopause creeping in. I returned to swimming, something I loved. But now I needed an environment to support that, too, so we built a pool.

This is what the PEO model looks like in real life: matching your home and habits to the person you are now.

Aging in Place Skills

When we talk about aging in place, it's easy to focus on big-picture decisions like home modifications or financial planning. But the real foundation of independence lies in the everyday skills we use without thinking.

Think about this morning. You likely got out of bed, used the toilet, showered, got dressed, made breakfast, did the dishes, threw in a load of laundry, and maybe fed the dog. These "small" things are actually complex skills we often take for granted.

OTs break these skills into:
- **ADLs** (Activities of Daily Living): bathing, dressing, toileting, eating.
- **IADLs** (Instrumental ADLs): cooking, shopping, cleaning, managing money.

Take grocery shopping, for example. Those breakfast ingredients didn't just magically appear in your fridge, right? You had to leave the house, drive, and navigate the store with enough stamina to walk and push a cart up and down the aisles. You needed visual scanning skills to find items, financial awareness to know how much to pay, and physical strength to load the groceries into your trunk. And even after you got home, you still needed the energy to unload everything and put it all away. That's not simple. It's a marathon of micro-skills.

The truth is, aging in place requires far more skills than most people realize. Beyond the basics of bathing and dressing, it includes everything from managing medications and paying bills online to mowing the lawn.

But life isn't just about getting through chores. It's also about holding onto the activities that bring us joy and purpose. That's why another key step is identifying the skills needed to maintain the things that matter most. For some, that might mean attending church each week or babysitting grandchildren. For others, it's a daily walk with a beloved dog or volunteering at the local hospital.

Aging in place means staying independent with these, and knowing when to get help. Thanks to the gig economy and delivery services, some IADLs are easier than ever to outsource: meal kits, housecleaners, Uber rides, and mobile pet grooming. But, like we discussed in Chapter 2, those services require financial planning.

So, here's your homework. Take some time to reflect:
- Which tasks bring me joy?
- Which ones do I want to keep doing myself?
- Which could I let go of?

I've worked with clients who never want to cook again, and others who *must* have their morning walk with their dog. For me? I'll work out an extra hour just to enjoy my beloved Canadian poutine—fries topped with cheese and gravy.

There are no wrong answers here. Being honest about what you value and what you're willing to do to keep it in your life is how you'll design a future that reflects who you are.

C3 | Practical Challenges of Aging in Place

The Evolving Homes® Model

I believe aging in place is about more than just staying home. It's about being well at home. This is the framework I developed to guide that thinking:

> **Cornerstone 1: Home Modification**:
> Are there tripping hazards in the home? Is it easy to move through your space? Could a walker or wheelchair fit if needed? A safe, accessible home is the foundation of aging in place.
>
> **Cornerstone 2: Physical Fitness**:
> Are you staying strong? Can you get up from the floor without help, carry groceries, or maintain balance in the shower? Strength, mobility, and endurance aren't just nice to have—they're essential to independence.
>
> **Cornerstone 3: Lifestyle Medicine**: Are you eating well, staying hydrated, sleeping enough, and maintaining routines that support your health? Aging in place is not possible if you're in and out of the hospital.
>
> **Cornerstone 4: Technology:** If you fall, will someone know? If you don't get out of bed, will someone be alerted? Are you socially connected? Technology can close the gap between safety and independence.

These cornerstones are interconnected. If one weakens, the others feel it, too. But when they work together? That's when people not only stay home, they *thrive* at home.

What This Looks Like in Real Life

- Sandy didn't want grab bars. But she *did* want to keep bathing alone. So, we installed a shampoo shelf that doubled as a support rail. It matched her tile, didn't scream "medical," and helped her feel elegant and safe. Six months later, she told me, "I love my spa shelf. I use it every day."
- Dennis hated the idea of "spying tech," but after a scary fall, we installed a radar sensor that would only alert his daughter if he didn't get out of bed by 9 a.m. He now calls it his "freedom detector."

Final Thoughts

Aging in place isn't just a goal. It's a lifestyle. It's the decision to stay in the place you love while continuing to do the things that make life meaningful.

In the chapters that follow, we'll take a deep dive into each of these cornerstones: what they mean, why they matter, and how you can start making small changes that build a safer, more empowered future at home.

I hope to inspire you, give you clear actions to take, and help you build a roadmap that works. Let's do this!

C3 | Practical Challenges of Aging in Place

Key Takeaways

- Aging in place means supporting your full routine, not just adding grab bars.
- OTs create custom plans to keep you independent at home.
- The PEO Model aligns your needs, space, and daily tasks.
- Every day activities get harder with age—plan ahead.
- Know what tasks matter most to you and protect them.
- Focus on the Four Cornerstones: Home Modification, Physical Fitness, Lifestyle Medicine, and Technology.
- Start early to build a home that supports how you want to live.

Chapter Four

What Is Universal Design?

Whether you've been updating each home you've lived in or are finally remodeling the one you plan to stay in, universal design should be your guiding principle.

Universal design is an approach to creating environments that are accessible, usable, and inclusive, right from the start. Rather than designing for your current needs and retrofitting later, universal design encourages you to plan for a wide range of users and situations from the beginning. It's about making spaces that work for everyone, regardless of age, size, or ability.

Universal Design Principles

Universal design may sound abstract, but it's actually about simple, thoughtful decisions that remove barriers without sacrificing aesthetics or functionality. Here are the core principles:

C4 | What Is Universal Design?

1. **Equitable** – Useful to people with diverse abilities.
   (Example: A ramp that benefits both wheelchair users and parents with strollers.)
2. **Flexibility in Use** – Accommodates a wide range of needs and preferences.
   (Example: Handheld showerheads or adjustable-height counters.)
3. **Simple and Intuitive** – Easy to understand, regardless of experience or ability.
   (Example: Intuitive controls and clearly marked signage.)
4. **Perceptible Information** – Communicates essential information effectively through multiple senses.
   (Example: Tactile paving combined with visual cues.)
5. **Tolerance for Error** – Minimizes hazards and reduces the risk of accidents.
   (Example: Appliances with automatic shut-off features.)
6. **Low Physical Effort** – Can be used efficiently and comfortably with minimal strain.
   (Example: Lever handles instead of traditional knobs.)
7. **Size and Space for Use** Provides adequate space for approach, reach, and movement.
   (Example: Wider doorways and clear, unobstructed pathways.)

These are the kinds of design choices that work for everyone, and they often go unnoticed because they just make sense.

Take curb cuts. They were designed for wheelchair users, but they help parents with strollers, travelers with rolling luggage, and delivery workers, too. Good design is universal.

In your home, it might look like:
- **No-step entries** that help toddlers, people with crutches, and aging adults alike.
- **Pull-down upper shelves** in cabinets so you don't need a step stool.

Age in Place or Find a New Space

- **Drawer-style base cabinets** to reduce bending and back strain.
- **Under-cabinet lighting** to brighten workspaces and eliminate shadows.
- **Matte countertop and floor finishes** that reduce glare for those with low vision.
- **Appliances placed at accessible heights** for people using wheelchairs or walkers.
- **Motion-sensor faucets and lighting** that require no twisting or searching in the dark.
- **Wider, intuitive hallways** that allow for side-by-side walking or mobility equipment.
- **Accessible microwave placement**—below the counter, not above the stove.

These choices serve a wide range of people: young families, aging adults, guests with mobility challenges, and even your future self. If you're already remodeling, why not make choices that serve you now and later?

Future-Proofing Your Home: Designing with Everyone in Mind

No one can predict exactly what they'll need in 30 years. But by keeping universal design in mind during routine updates, you're making the most efficient use of your time and money. You're creating a space that can adapt with you, without having to start over every time life changes.

I've applied this mindset in my own home. When our kids got older, my husband and I decided to renovate the kitchen. We knew the 30-inch doorway and a two-inch drop between rooms had to go. I'd already seen too many scraped knees and near falls. So, leveling the flooring became non-negotiable and worth the $2,500 price tag.

We didn't just widen the doorway, we took out the whole wall. It created a seamless 42-inch opening that felt open and inviting and also gave me room to install a professional-grade stove someday. (Eating is my #1 hobby; cooking is a close second.)

C4 | What Is Universal Design?

During the remodel, I was intentional about every choice: balancing safety, independence, and long-term usability. To help reduce common causes of falls, I opted for drawer-style base cabinets, minimizing the need to bend forward for extended periods. I also prioritized my kids' independence by placing the microwave below the countertop instead of above the stove, making it easier and safer for them to use. Every detail reflected ease and adaptability—from motion-sensor lights inside drawers to a four-door refrigerator with a convertible compartment that can function as either a fridge or freezer. I reimagined where everything should go, placing items in locations I thought would be more accessible, both now and if my needs change in the future.

And that's the thing—it wasn't just about me when I leveled the kitchen and repositioned the appliances. If my teenage son were to break his leg and needed a wheelchair for a few months, he'd need smooth, level flooring to move from room to room. He'd also need appliances that are easy to reach and intuitively placed.

As an occupational therapist, I think constantly about how environments support independence and function. That's why I designed the lowest pull-out drawer in my tower cabinet to include an electric outlet, so the kids could handle their own spills without needing help. The cords stay tucked away neatly, reducing fall risks and keeping the space safe for everyone.

And universal design doesn't stop in the kitchen.

What about the front entrance? If a friend shows up with a stroller or your dad needs a walker, can they get in? I've had clients tell me that their own family can't visit because their home isn't accessible. It's a powerful reminder that thoughtful design isn't just about convenience, it's about connection and inclusion.

The beauty of universal design is that it supports multi-generational living—not just across different family members, but across all the versions of ourselves as we grow, age, and change. Design decisions like wider doors and no-step entries aren't about disability;

they're about inclusion. They make your home usable across generations and life stages.

Visitability: Because Everyone Deserves a Way In

Visitability means that anyone who visits your home can enter and use the bathroom without a struggle. We baby-proof for toddlers. Why not "people-proof" for everyone else?

Even delivery drivers benefit. I once lived in a third-floor walk-up and watched a poor guy wrestle a fridge up three flights of stairs. He sourly remarked that the only way it was coming back down was through a window. That's the cost of not planning ahead.

Thoughtful updates, like no-step entries and wider doors, aren't just for your future self. They create a more welcoming, flexible home for guests, friends, and aging loved ones.

When you're making updates to your house, consider incorporating small, thoughtful changes over the years to improve accessibility. These design choices add little cost during renovation but can be extremely costly and messy when done as a retrofit.

Lastly, these thoughtful changes don't just benefit you and your family. They make your home more welcoming for friends and guests, too. It's an investment in visitability, a concept that prioritizes convenience and inclusion for everyone who walks through your door. And when done well, it's almost invisible. It simply works.

ADA vs. Universal Design: Why ADA Rules Don't Fit Your House

Many people assume they should "follow ADA guidelines" when remodeling, but the ADA was written for public spaces, not personal homes. ADA bathrooms are one-size-fits-all solutions meant to

C4 | What Is Universal Design?

accommodate a wide range of extremes, from individuals under 5 feet tall to over 6 feet 6 inches. But that's not what you need in your home. It's like hearing, *"This one-size-fits-all t-shirt is going to fit me perfectly and make me look amazing!"* Probably not.

Your home should be customized for the people who live there. It should reflect your habits, your routines, and your goals, not some federal checklist. Our highest level of function happens when the environment is tailored to support who you are today and what you need to do. That kind of support is highly specific and deeply personal.

That's why I always say: building an ADA bathroom should not be the goal. You're not designing for the general public. You're designing for the small number of people who use that space every single day.

The goal is to create an environment that supports your unique lifestyle. That's where an occupational therapist can help. We ask the awkward questions—like how you get on and off the toilet or manage in the shower—and design with empathy, dignity, and discretion. We're trained to talk through these deeply personal details with empathy and discretion.

There's no one-size-fits-all, no absolute "right" or "wrong." The only important question is: What works best for you? And when that kind of honest insight is part of the design process, it becomes much easier to create a home that works with you, not against you.

Final Thoughts

Nearly 90 percent of adults over 50 want to age in place. Yet fewer than five percent of U.S. homes are even considered mobility-friendly and less than one percent are fully accessible.[ix]

That means most homes will need modifications. And those updates are much easier and cheaper to make if you start early and spread them out over time.

The good news? You don't have to do everything at once. Planning ahead takes effort but it's one of the most meaningful

Age in Place or Find a New Space

investments you can make. By making thoughtful changes over time, you spread out the cost, reduce disruption, and lighten the emotional weight of future transitions. Every step you take now is a gift to your future self and possibly someone else down the road.

Whether you stay in your home forever or move closer to family down the line, the changes you make today increase the availability of accessible housing in your community.

Your thoughtful upgrades might someday benefit someone else who needs them more than you ever did. And that's a legacy worth investing in.

C4 | What Is Universal Design?

Key Takeaways

- Design your home to be accessible for all ages and abilities from the start.
- Choose flexible features like adjustable counters and handheld fixtures that adapt over time.
- Universal design can be both beautiful and highly functional.
- Wide doorways and level floors make movement safer and easier for everyone.
- Thoughtful layouts and appliance placement support daily independence.
- Focus on what works for your lifestyle, not just ADA standards.
- Every inclusive choice you make helps your home welcome more people.

Chapter Five

Why People Resist—and How to Gently Shift the Mindset

One of the most common phrases I hear from adult children is that their parents are in denial of physical changes.

"I'm not losing my hearing. The TV was too loud, so I couldn't hear you."

"That towel rack was loose already. I only hold onto it because it's there."

"I don't want any of that stuff. That's for old people."

It's a frustrating experience for family members who just want to help, especially when offered solutions fall on deaf ears (pun intended). However, all kidding aside, what can be done in this situation?

For me, I've found that conversations flow better if you ask for more clarity, approach the problem with genuine curiosity and a heartfelt desire to understand.

C5 | Why People Resist—and How to Gently Shift the Mindset

Denial of Physical Changes

As we've discussed, it can be incredibly difficult to visualize your future self, especially when there's a disconnect between who you were and who you are now. I've found that I struggle with this a little less, thanks to the wonderful patients I've had the privilege of working with over the past 27 years.

When I worked as an occupational therapist in inpatient rehab, my day started early—often by 6:30 a.m. on the patient floors. In OT, our focus is on helping people regain independence in everyday tasks like getting dressed, brushing their teeth, and combing their hair. It's always been my favorite part of the job, because I loved the quiet, meaningful conversations I'd have with older adults as they got ready to face the day.

While they worked on the skills needed to dress independently, which often required frequent breaks due to shortness of breath or fatigue, I had the privilege of hearing fascinating adventures of their younger selves and witnessing the excitement on their faces as they vividly brought each story to life in great detail.

We would then get up from the bed, walk to the bathroom, and without fail, almost every patient would look in the mirror to comb their hair and remark, "I have no idea who that old person is in the mirror. I feel 25 inside."

The reason I share this story is to show that people aren't in denial on purpose. That sense of youthfulness in the mind—the same spark you see in their eyes—often doesn't register the physical aging happening in the body. When you combine that with constant marketing messages that glorify youth and frame aging as something negative, it's easy to understand why someone might see a helpful product on TV and not recognize it as relevant to their own life.

Fear of Loss

Many patients have shared that their fear isn't installing the grab bar or removing the throw rug itself. It's what those changes represent. They

Age in Place or Find a New Space

worry that the moment they agree to install one or remove the other, it will trigger an avalanche of changes, marking the start of a long, downward spiral. To them, it feels like the beginning of a list of losses, simply because they're getting older.

In my opinion, there's absolutely no reason to say that stairs are bad, rugs are dangerous, or wheelchairs are inherently good. Or that being over 65 means you're suddenly banned from climbing a ladder ever again.

And there is a belief out there that assumes aging is a predictable downhill slide that occurs the same way with everyone. First, it's the grab bar, then it's the shower seat, next is a walker, and then you'll be in a wheelchair.

When aging is framed as a slow surrender of everything you love, it's no wonder people resist it. When every recommendation sounds like, "You can't do that anymore," the natural reaction is to push back. No one wants to feel like their identity is being chipped away one safety feature at a time. Unfortunately, that fear is often reinforced by misinformation online or casual, offhand comments like, "Well, you're not a spring chicken anymore."

But here's the truth: there are many kinds of 65-year-olds in this world. It's not fair or helpful to compare an active, healthy 65-year-old to someone the same age with multiple chronic conditions and limited mobility. Age alone tells us very little. That's why it's so important to reject one-size-fits-all solutions.

Instead, approach each person as a unique individual and build a plan based on their specific needs, values, and goals. Too often, people view aging with a sense of resignation, when in reality, aging is what you make of it. You are an active participant in shaping your future. The bricks you lay today become the path you walk tomorrow. And the direction you take? That's entirely up to you.

C5 | Why People Resist—and How to Gently Shift the Mindset

Avoidance of the Issues

My friend, Cathy, who is an elder care attorney, once shared that her clients often admitted to avoiding her office because of an irrational belief that if they prepared their will, they would soon need it.

Making plans to prepare for the future can feel like giving up or admitting defeat. "Carol, the reason I'm avoiding my daughter's calls because she keeps bugging me to go on a tour of a retirement community. They are trying to put me out to pasture and I'm not having it!!"

So much resistance is due to assumptions and a lack of perspective. By stepping into the other person's shoes, you can find a way to approach with compassion, and mindsets can be changed.

In this case, the daughter is feeling anxious after the last hospitalization and wants to start looking at options to get a sense of what feels right for her mom. She wants to have a plan to decrease the stress that comes from having to make sudden decisions.

My patient is feeling insecure about her future and perceives her daughter's nudge as a loss of control over her life. She doesn't want to have that conversation, so she avoids it. Understandably, her daughter gets frustrated. And then she gets frustrated. And then they don't talk. And then she has a bad fall. And then she ends up in the only community that had availability, which isn't a good fit.

Ouch.

Preparing for the future is about staying in control and not waiting until things spiral out of it. It means making decisions while you have the mental space to thoughtfully evaluate your options. You have the clarity, the calm, and the confidence to keep an open mind knowing that, in the end, you hold the veto power.

What did I say to that patient? "Your daughter loves you and just wants the reassurance that there's a plan, whether that means staying at home or moving to a community. Be brave. Go on the tour. Gather information. Do it for your future self and as a gift of peace of mind for your daughter."

Too Many Decisions

One of the biggest obstacles I see when it comes to home modifications is what I call *Big-Ticket Paralysis by Analysis*. This happens when people get stuck, sometimes for months, trying to decide on something like the location or color of a grab bar or shower fixture. And I get it. Once you drill into tile, you are pretty much committed. But you can't let that fear run your life.

That's exactly why I developed an integrated system of products and design strategies—to take the guesswork and hesitation out of the process. This system can transform a standard tub into a stylish, walk-in shower in under a week. It's the ideal solution for someone coming home from the hospital who needs a functional space quickly but also values beauty and personal choice.

But even with a good system in place, there are lessons you only learn through experience.

During my research, I fell in love with an innovative shower system from Home Depot: imported from China, beautifully designed, and perfectly aligned with my vision and budget. But my excitement was short-lived. The moment my plumber saw it, he warned me I'd regret installing it. I had been so mesmerized by the look of it that I hadn't even thought to consider the weight. The support hinges were made of flimsy metal, and I knew he was right. Over time, the lightweight metal would likely bend or break, leaving me stuck replacing the entire fixture again and again. Worse, since the holes would already be drilled, I'd be locked into that brand and placement, unless I wanted to re-tile the entire wall.

What did I learn from that experience? Keep it simple. I now follow the KISS method (Keep It Simple, Stupid). Whenever I start feeling anxious about a decision, I prioritize the simplest version to lower my commitment stress. I also choose fixtures with flexibility, ones I can easily switch out later without major renovations.

Ultimately, I chose to do a simple, external shower fixture that only had 2 attachment points to drill. The brand came with a 10-year warranty which gave me confidence in the durability of their product. It

C5 | Why People Resist—and How to Gently Shift the Mindset

was also available in multiple colors so that if I wanted to change the look later, I had options. So, my advice is to scale things back and just do the parts you know for sure.

Bathroom renovations don't have to be all or nothing. As you saw in the example above, the only change I made was to the tub area. In hospital-to-home situations, I almost always leave the toilet, sink, and flooring untouched. Why is that? Because, in most cases, there are other ways to manage the tasks that happen there at no additional cost—they can brush their teeth at the kitchen sink and use a bedside commode for toileting if needed. But bathing? That's a different story.

There really aren't many good alternatives aside from what my military patients jokingly call "spit baths." And let's be honest, that's not the same thing at all. When patients finally get to take a real shower after a week of sponge bathing, they don't want to get out. I've had people tell me it feels *heavenly*—the warm water hitting their face and back, the simple joy of rinsing off and feeling truly clean again.

So, let go of the assumption that you "have to" renovate the entire bathroom all at once to make it worthwhile. Don't let that mindset be the reason you stay stuck and make no progress at all.

Longtime Homeowners

One of the biggest reasons people resist change, especially later in life, is the sheer emotional and logistical weight of "stuff." Many older adults have lived in their homes for 30 years or more. Facing the idea of moving or even just tidying up can be overwhelming. It's not just about objects; it's about memories, identity, and tough choices. Where do you begin when everything feels important? Sorting through a lifetime of belongings is mentally and emotionally exhausting. For many, it's easier to leave Pandora's box sealed, promising themselves they'll deal with it another day. But that day, of course, never comes.

The best way I've found to generate momentum is by bringing in a neutral third party. Set up the service, pay the invoice, and then graciously step back. This approach helps families preserve their emotional bonds and focus on meaningful conversations, not arguments over keeping mismatched Tupperware or tossing boxes of school projects.

One of my favorite referrals is to a professional organizer. These individuals act like coaches: empathetic yet firm, gently guiding clients through the emotional process of letting go. They provide structure, accountability, and encouragement. Over time, the overwhelming becomes manageable. Again and again, I hear clients say, *"I can't believe how much lighter I feel."*

Another go-to referral is a handyman who can help tackle deferred maintenance—things like fixing loose floorboards, changing light fixtures, or clearing gutters. I also suggest practical safety upgrades like installing a second handrail or moving boxes out of walkways.

These services are typically well-received because they reduce stress for everyone, regardless of age. I often recommend organizing or handyman session packages as holiday gifts because they're thoughtful, useful, and instead of adding clutter, they help eliminate it.

What I appreciate most about working with a professional organizer is that it keeps the homeowner engaged. Decisions are made with purpose, not haste. It's a respectful, empowering process, nothing like the emotional trauma of watching your treasured belongings being tossed into a dumpster.

Decluttering does take effort but it's free, and it's one of the most cost-effective ways to prevent falls. To guide the process, I always recommend starting in two of the most common areas for falls, the bedroom and the bathroom. We'll talk in more detail in the next few chapters.

Not Enough Money

I hear this a lot, and it's a valid concern, especially if they're living on a fixed income. One of the best first steps is to involve their financial

C5 | Why People Resist—and How to Gently Shift the Mindset

advisor early in the process. That professional has a full view of an older adult's financial health and can help assess what's actually affordable. Sometimes, hearing it from a trusted third party is just what is needed.

I've also learned from years of doing home assessments that not all financial resistance is really about money. More than once, an adult child has pulled me aside to say, "Don't listen to them. They can afford it. They just don't want to spend it." I have also heard from older clients, "It's not that I can't afford the changes, I just don't want them." It's not always about the cost; sometimes, it's more about control, comfort, or fear of change.

So, the question is, what mindset shift is required to see home modifications as something that decreases their stress, increases their freedom or saves them money in the long run?

My experience is that the answer lies in identifying what that person sees as valuable and what would motivate that person to make those changes.

People are motivated by incentives, so while it can feel daunting to invest $30,000 or more in a bathroom renovation, there are smart ways to reframe it as a decision that can save you money in the long run.

Try Before You Buy

You know what else costs about as much as a bathroom remodel? A car. And how do we make peace with that kind of big purchase? We test drive it. We take it around the block, see how it feels because it's a big investment, and we want to know it's the right fit. Now, how many times have you tried a feature in a friend's car, like heated seats or a backup camera, and thought, "Okay, I need this in my next car?" Why does this happen? Because you don't know what you don't know until you've experienced it.

The same thing happens with bathroom remodels. I once had a client in her 80s, living independently, with no mobility issues, and who had never considered home modification until a family reunion cruise

Age in Place or Find a New Space

changed her perspective. The cruise line had assigned her to an accessible cabin, complete with grab bars, a roll-in shower, and plenty of space to move around. What surprised her most wasn't how it looked, but how *easy* everything felt. The layout, the safety features, and the thoughtful design just worked better. She didn't have to think twice about balance, wet floors, or reaching for things. When she got home, she told me, "I would never have agreed to make those kinds of changes, but now that I've tried it, I want the same thing in my house!" Sometimes, it just takes one good experience to shift your whole perspective.

In other cases, it takes your wife of 30 years to help you see a better way. My patient and her husband were high school sweethearts and so adorable together. As many wives do, she worried about him needing to step over the tub to take a shower. As many husbands do, he felt that he did not need support in his bathroom.

Despite the protests, she went ahead and ordered matching grab bars for his bathroom, and I sized them for his much taller height, so he'd be functional and comfortable. We also added a shampoo shelf grab bar to keep his toiletries from slipping off the edge of the tub—no more bending over or stepping on a dropped bottle. And we installed a towel bar grab bar, giving him another safe handhold for getting in and out of the tub.

Wouldn't you know that when I did a follow up visit to their home, he couldn't stop raving about how much he loved the grab bars, how much more secure he felt with them in and how wonderful it was that because of the color contrast, he could find the grab bars even with soap in his eyes!

For my clients who hate waste and value efficiency, I focus on the long-term benefits, like improved resale value and the opportunity to enjoy the upgrades *now*, instead of waiting until a crisis forces the issue. I also point out how much harder it is to retrofit a space later. Once the tile is drilled or plumbing is set, mistakes can be costly, and that tends to get people's attention.

C5 | Why People Resist—and How to Gently Shift the Mindset

For those hesitant to spend money on grab bars, I shift the conversation toward priorities. Grab bars might be a financial investment, but they're a *passive* solution. Exercise, on the other hand, is cheap, but it requires consistent effort. So, the real question becomes: *what do you want to invest in?* There's no wrong answer, only what matters most to you.

Some people may dislike exercise, but when they realize that staying strong could delay or even reduce the need for paid care down the line, many begin to warm up to the idea of doing those sit-ups and push-ups after all.

The key is to stay curious, be supportive, and create space for honest conversations. When we respect autonomy while gently helping someone weigh risks and benefits, it often leads to better, more lasting outcomes for everyone.

Suction Grab Bars Are a Gateway Drug

Suction grab bars are not the bad guy. I've come to think of them as one of the most helpful tools in gently guiding people toward safer, more accessible choices in their homes.

Many of my clients will immediately be on guard the minute they even smell a conversation about grab bars brewing. For them, bars symbolize aging, weakness, and decline. So, when someone flat-out refuses to even consider installing one, my strategy is to ask if they would be willing to let me put up a suction grab bar instead. These little exposures give my clients a chance to experience how much more secure they feel with just a minor change. Many times, when I would return for a follow-up visit, I would get a reluctant "humph" as they admit, "Okay, maybe it was a little helpful."

I have also discovered over the years that the suction grab bar is my favorite MacGyver-like multi-tool. They not only protect your joints by using better body mechanics, but the normal use of them in everyday

Age in Place or Find a New Space

life also helps older adults see grab bars as helpful and just a smarter way to accomplish a task that has nothing to do with aging.

One of my most common uses outside the bathroom is to put a suction grab bar on the door of the dryer. This can help people with hand weakness, as it's so much easier to open a door if you have a proper handle instead of trying to get enough leverage by only using the tips of your fingers. Stackable dryers, a great space-saving solution, often pose additional challenges because of their height and the required shoulder-level motion. This can be difficult to manage for older adults, particularly given the high prevalence of rotator cuff tears in this age group.

One study found a 22 percent prevalence of full-thickness rotator cuff tears in adults over 60, with that number rising to over 50 percent in those over 80.[x] These tears are typically the result of a degenerative process that is a natural part of aging, but the loss of range of motion, increased pain, and weakness during overhead activities has a direct impact on daily function, making even routine tasks difficult.

Another everyday place where I often recommend using a suction grab bar is on sliding glass doors. These doors can be surprisingly difficult to open, especially for older adults with rotator cuff injuries. The effort required to operate them can make accessing outdoor living spaces uncomfortable, limiting a person's ability to enjoy the places they love most.

Once again, this isn't just a solution for older adults. I have a suction grab bar on my own patio door—not because I'm injured, but for joint protection reasons. So many people suffer from arthritis in their fingers in later years, and that pain can rob them of the joy found in their favorite hobbies. The key to avoiding this fate is to get into the habit early of using the largest, strongest joints. like your shoulder or elbow, whenever possible, so your smaller joints can be preserved for the tasks they're best at, like fine motor activities. Whether it's buttoning a shirt, sewing, or using utensils, your fingers deserve to be protected so that your function is protected.

C5 | Why People Resist—and How to Gently Shift the Mindset

I also use suction grab bars to teach someone how to ease themselves into the tub and provide light support for getting back up. While they're not meant to bear full weight, they can offer just enough assistance to improve confidence and safety during the movement.

Suction grab bars fall off shower walls because of poor suction caused by uneven tile surfaces, grout lines, or the natural curve of the wall. But bathtubs are a different story. Their smooth, flat surfaces provide a much more reliable seal for temporary use.

Is it perfect? No. But is it helpful to show how a permanent grab bar might make life easier? Absolutely.

What I've found is that the constant maintenance required, like reminding someone, "Every time you take a shower, you'll need to budget a few extra minutes to do a safety check on the bar", often becomes the tipping point. The reality is that suction grab bars are unpredictable. You can't always trust them to hold your weight, and that uncertainty becomes inconvenient at best and unsafe at worst.

That's usually when the light bulb goes off. They realize it's more of a hassle to constantly check and re-secure a suction bar than to just install a permanent one. And the best part? They aren't taking the action because I talked them into it. They do it because they have experienced the limitations firsthand and made the decision themselves. A small shift, but a powerful one.

Grab Bar Stigma

Many people resist installing grab bars because they wrongly assume they are only for the frail and weak. This assumption is why grab bars are in dire need of a rebranding strategy. Grab bars are for everyone. In my opinion, they should be a standard bathroom safety feature because they prevent injury.

When I get doubtful looks, I like to tell the story of John Glenn, America's first astronaut to orbit the Earth (with no injury more than a skinned knuckle) and fighter pilot in the South Pacific. At the age of 42, at the peak of his physical fitness, John slipped in his bathroom, and he hit his head on the edge of the bathtub hard enough to cause a traumatic brain injury (TBI). His persistent dizziness and balance issues forced him to withdraw from the US Senatorial race in 1964. He wasn't old or aging but the consequences of that fall impacted his ability to live the life he had imagined for himself. Bathroom safety helps everyone be their best selves.

Like Seatbelts in a Car

The other thing I like to point out is that grab bars are no different than the seatbelts in your car. They are there to decrease the risk of serious injury or death in unforeseen circumstances and are a non-negotiable safety feature. Ninety-nine percent of the time, they are never needed, but when they are, those seatbelts save lives. If you had an easy solution that you could do now, that could prevent serious injury later, why *wouldn't* you plan to put it in and use it?

Do It for the Grandchildren

Older adults aren't the only ones who benefit from secure handholds. A close friend of mine was babysitting her grandchild one evening when, during bath time, the wiggling toddler slipped and hit his head on the tub faucet. Instead of settling in for bedtime stories and snuggles, she found herself rushing to the emergency room, where her grandson was diagnosed with a concussion.

In my experience, older adults might hesitate when it comes to spending money on themselves, but when it comes to protecting their grandchildren, they don't think twice. *"I don't need grab bars for myself, but my ball-of-energy grandson does—so I'm going to put them in."* When you reframe upgrades, like adding grab bars, non-slip surfaces, or better lighting, as ways to create a safer, more welcoming space for visiting loved ones, things feel different. Suddenly, the conversation isn't

C5 | Why People Resist—and How to Gently Shift the Mindset

about them aging. It's about being a protective grandparent, a thoughtful host, and a person who's planning ahead for everyone's comfort. The best part of this is that they get to enjoy the benefits of those same changes on the other 350 days a year when the grandkids *aren't* visiting.

And speaking of children, let's not forget that middle-aged adults also benefit from grab bars. I learned that firsthand.

Back when I was working as a home health clinician, I had a suction grab bar that I'd bring with me to show patients how a grab bar could make it easier to get in and out of the tub. It also helped us figure out the ideal height and placement before committing to a permanent installation.

For convenience, I stored it in my kids' bathroom, stuck to the wall so I wouldn't lose track of it. My kids were little at the time, and my husband often handled bath duty. He'd sit on the edge of the tub with his feet in the water while washing them. One night, I heard a loud "Aaugh! Carol! Where did the grab bar go?"

I didn't realize he'd been using the grab bar for balance while washing the kids until that day when I let a patient borrow it overnight. Sometimes, the clearest sign that a home modification is helpful is when it's unexpectedly gone and you find yourself missing it.

Unaware of Beautiful Options

Another common reason people resist making changes in their homes is that they don't know options for beautiful accessibility exist. They assume their personally curated homes will begin to look and feel like hospitals if they allow people to "make it safer." It doesn't have to be like that.

What you see at big box stores is just a small window into the options out there. There are many gorgeous designs that you would be happy to put into your spaces. So many times, people have walked into a bathroom I've designed and asked, "Where are the grab bars?" because these days, many hand holds can be hidden in plain sight, multi-functional fixtures. You can buy a combo grab bar/towel bar, a grab bar/toilet paper holder, or a grab bar/corner shelf from many different manufacturers.

"Beautiful accessibility" is the phrase I like to use to describe leveraging solutions with an ideal balance of beauty and function. It may seem unimportant or even counterintuitive to prioritize beauty over function, but calm feelings are actually produced in the brain when exposed to beauty. When combined with feelings of security elicited by purposefully located safety measures, everyone wins.

In my experience, homeowners who are presented with choices that resonate with their personal styles and preferences are much more likely to integrate safety measures into their environments and regain harmony among the three PEO Model spheres. Aesthetics can be one obstacle to change, but perceptions can also play an influencing role.

Improve Resale Value

Installing grab bars is often viewed as an unnecessary expense by older adults. One discussion I like to have is talking about how adding beautiful safety features can increase your home's value and marketability, making your house attractive for buyers of all age groups. A study focusing on the Portland, Oregon, area found that converting a bathroom to meet universal design standards could recoup approximately 60.8 percent of the renovation costs upon resale.[xi] A 2024 cost versus value report indicated that in the Florida area, 49.5 percent of construction costs are recouped when outfitting a bathroom with universal design elements.[xii]

When you re-frame the expense as an investment in the value of your home, it makes it much easier to say yes to beautiful grab bars. One of my favorite places to start is to show clients unique products like wave-shaped grab bars or stylistic dual-purpose, toilet paper grab bars that can add visual interest to the space. "It's the jewelry of the bathroom!" one client commented after I showed her the possibilities.

C5 | Why People Resist—and How to Gently Shift the Mindset

Use Objective Data to Start a Conversation

One of the most powerful things we can do in conversations related to change is to take the drama out of it. When emotions are high, I find it helps to rely on objective data instead of emotional assumptions.

"I'm just trying to keep you safe!" feels like control. Instead, saying, "Here's what we know. Let's look at it together." For example, instead of jumping into a heated debate about what someone should or shouldn't do, we might lay out the facts: "This is what your current home costs to maintain. Here's the estimate for renovations. Here's what a similar home next door is going for, and here's what it would take to make it accessible."

It's just information. No judgment. No pressure. Just clarity.

It's the same approach when it applies to safety. When families sit down to talk about whether it's still safe for someone to live alone, it can feel deeply personal, almost like an accusation. "Dad, we're worried you can't manage living on your own anymore" can be hard to hear.

But what if the conversation started with something more grounded, like data from a month of sensor tracking? What if you could gently say, "Dad, the stove was left on three times this month. Does that concern you?" Now it's not about blaming or forcing a decision. It's about inviting them into the process, with compassion and respect.

That's how you create a space where everyone can breathe a little easier. It's not about making someone feel bad, it's about saying, "I care about you. I want us both to sleep well at night." It's a shared understanding that we all live with risk. We all do things that aren't 100 percent safe—whether that's leaving the stove on or having French fries for dinner. The point is to give people the freedom to decide which risks they're willing to live with, and which ones can be planned for together.

You'll Be in Their Shoes Someday: Reframing the Conversation

The way you have these conversations makes all the difference in how well the message is received. It helps to try to see things through your loved ones' eyes and recognize that someday, you'll likely be in their shoes too. That kind of empathy softens the conversation for everyone. I try to connect the dots in a way that helps families relate to one another.

For example, adult children can better understand their parents' experiences by remembering that they themselves have also changed over time. It's likely that adult children have also faced things that were hard to give up as they moved from the boundless energy of their 20s to the popping joints of their 50s. That moment of "Oh… I get it now" can open the door to real connection.

Too often, people view "my life" as separate from "my parent's aging," when it's more accurate to realize it's all part of the same journey—just different roles at different stages and all asking the same big questions. When you help people see themselves in their parents, they stop trying to push and spend more time inviting them into a conversation about how to make life easier, safer, and more fulfilling.

The Answer Is Somewhere in the Middle

Some people look at spaces purely from a physical perspective (what's accessible, what's code-compliant) because it's easy, it's transactional. Emotions are messy and hard to navigate. They're rarely black and white. And the truth is, most people either don't know how to handle that complexity or would rather avoid it altogether.

Fortunately, occupational therapists are trained in both physical rehabilitation and mental health. Our profession is a unique blend of art and science, and we often rely on what's called the "therapeutic use of self"—using our own life experiences and insights as part of the healing process. In many ways, we're part life coach, part rehab specialist,

C5 | Why People Resist—and How to Gently Shift the Mindset

helping people not just recover but reconnect with what gives their lives meaning and purpose.

This is where occupational therapists shine. We're trained to find that balance between safety and the meaningful elements that give a person's life richness and identity.

For example, many of my patients are former military. When you're privileged enough to work in someone's home, you get a front-row seat to what truly matters to them. You start to see how they've carefully curated a comforting environment filled with memories, often including items brought back from tours of duty, like antique rugs or delicate end tables. These pieces aren't just furniture; they're symbols of history, pride, and personal meaning. Our role is to respect that while gently guiding changes that support both safety and dignity.

I try to make sure that my patients know that my goal isn't to take things away. It's to help them understand the trade-offs and make purposeful decisions. I present the pros and cons based on my knowledge and training, and then I let them decide what makes the most sense to incorporate into their lives. I will push to let go of something when the fall risk is significant and the problem doesn't hold much sentimental value. But for things that *do* matter, I'll work with them to dig deep for a solution to make it work for them. This team approach makes it easier to compromise on the right balance of safety and risk for everyone.

Six Inches Is Still Progress: The Power of Tiny Wins

One of the places where people get stuck is thinking that solutions must be all-or-nothing. A useful skill we learn in our training is the ability to break an activity down into small chunks. This decreases the shutdown that people get when they are overwhelmed, and it makes the activity feel more attainable and reasonable. It's OK to start wherever you are.

What this looks like in real life is by me asking the question, "What's one itty-bitty, small step you would feel comfortable taking that can move you in the direction that you want to be going?" Sometimes that answer is as small as, "Well, I'll consider letting you move that glass table off to the side, but no more than 6 inches, OK?" And you know what my response is? "Awesome! Sounds like a plan!"

Overcoming inertia is the biggest challenge for anyone trying to make changes in their lives. This is why taking baby steps, even if it's an ant-sized baby step, is good enough for me. We are building trust with our agreement. If one week later, the request is to put it back, it goes back. When I do what I promise, without judgment, they know they are the ones in control of this bus. This is how momentum is built in my experience. You start small and move forward from there. If you get stuck, move on. I might focus on a different change in a different part of the house. And maybe come back to that glass table in a month. If the trend is moving forward, no matter how slow it might be, celebrate that it's moving!

Final Thoughts

As you have seen, aging in place is not a one-size-fits-all experience and is definitely not a solo sport.

It's a journey on a shifting foundation so staying flexible and open to whatever comes your way is key. Everyone responds positively when they see that their plan is personalized and that their priorities are front and center.

When we feel heard, we feel safe enough to have a heart-to-heart discussion about what is really going on beneath the surface.

Find out what matters. Discover what options are available to make sure that the things that matter the most in your life stay in your life.

Once you know what you want, it's easy to reverse-engineer your life to make choices that will get you to where you want to be. When there is a plan, everyone feels better. Promise.

So, let's get to work. We are going to dig into what those options are to support the Four Pillars of Aging in Place in the next few chapters.

C5 | Why People Resist—and How to Gently Shift the Mindset

Key Takeaways

- People often resist changes because they don't see themselves as aging.
- Fear of loss and identity drives much of the hesitation.
- Avoidance stems from anxiety, not ignorance—approach with compassion.
- Too many choices can stall action—keep solutions simple and flexible.
- Decluttering and maintenance can be emotional—bring in neutral helpers.
- Money objections are often about control, not affordability.
- Trying safety features firsthand can change minds.
- Suction grab bars can ease people into permanent solutions.
- Reframe upgrades as beautiful, protective, and beneficial for everyone.
- Start small, personalize the approach, and always lead with empathy.

Chapter Six

Home Modification

In the last few chapters, we have talked about the importance of starting early to build positive habits, doing research to know what you want, and discussing the challenges that come with aging in place, both physically and emotionally.

Now, it's time to talk about what features are important to consider when preparing your home for aging in place.

This chapter follows the room-by-room assessment that I would normally do if I were at your home today. I'll talk about what my *#otbrain* is thinking and what I'm looking for as I walk through your spaces.

My goal is to teach you how to see your home through my eyes, so you can understand the basics and then personalize it—adding all the herbs and seasonings that make it uniquely yours. A home assessment is about identifying potential fall risks and exploring ways to reduce them. I'll walk you through what to look for and share some of my favorite solutions for common challenges. Are you ready? Let's get started!

C6 | Home Modification

Exterior Accessibility

My home assessment doesn't begin at the front door. It begins the moment I pull into the driveway. I'm already scanning the big picture: the condition of the driveway, the layout of the yard, the quality of lighting, and how the home presents itself from the outside.

Some of the biggest red flags appear before I even step inside the house. I might observe cracks in the driveway that could be tripped on, loose gravel that could affect balance, or uneven pavers along the front path—all potential fall hazards. I'm also thinking about emergency access: What would happen if you needed help right now? Could a paramedic find your house? Could they get a stretcher through your entryway?

I recently visited a home with a beautiful winding path to the front door that was very pretty, but only 26" wide with uneven flagstones, making it a trip hazard and likely almost impossible to self-propel with a walker or wheelchair. The homeowner admitted she hadn't noticed since she always entered through the garage. My vote is that her friends, family, delivery drivers, and emergency responders have noticed.

What I'm Looking For

- **Driveway condition:** Is it smooth, level, and free of potholes or loose rock?
- **House number visibility:** Can emergency services or guests find your home easily?
- **Exterior lighting:** Are walkways and entries lit up enough to navigate after dark?
- **Shrubbery and landscaping:** Are bushes trimmed back to avoid crowding walkways?
- **Walkway width and surface:** Is the path 36–48" wide? Is it non-slip and level?

Age in Place or Find a New Space

> - **Emergency access:** Could a stretcher or large equipment get into the home quickly?
> - **Garage/front door entry:** Are either of these accessible in a wheelchair or during temporary injury?

Quick DIY Wins

- ☐ Trim hedges and remove overgrown plants that narrow walkways.
- ☐ Use a contrasting color of mulch or gravel to draw attention to the edges of the walkway.
- ☐ Add solar-powered path lighting.
- ☐ Use outdoor-rated, high-contrast paint to mark out areas you need to pay extra attention to.
- ☐ Secure loose pavers or replace gravel paths with solid surfaces.
- ☐ Make your house number more visible from the street—reflective, high-contrast numbers are best. Consider relocating if you will need to constantly trim shrubs to maintain visibility.
- ☐ Add a Hide-A-Key or emergency-access lockbox for caregivers or EMS.

When to Call a Pro

- √ Replace uneven or broken concrete in the driveway or walk path.
- √ Install motion-sensor floodlights to illuminate the house number.
- √ Expand narrow paths to at least 36", ideally 48", for mobility device use.
- √ Have a landscaper evaluate whether adjusting the slope of the ground around your home could allow for a "ramp-scape"—a gradual sidewalk integrated into the landscaping that functions as a ramp while blending seamlessly with the outdoor design.

C6 | Home Modification

Homeowner/Caregiver Self-Audit

- Is the driveway smooth and free of potholes or shifting gravel?
- Is the house number clearly visible from the street, day and night?
- Are shrubs or bushes crowding walkways?
- Can someone safely walk from the driveway to the door using a walker or cane?
- Is there a clear, step-free route into the home?
- Could emergency personnel roll a stretcher into the house without obstruction?

#OTBrain Insight

Every second counts in an emergency. Your home's exterior tells a story about safety, maintenance, and readiness. A well-lit, accessible path isn't just welcoming, it could be lifesaving.

・・・

Connect with Your Local Fire Station

Another often overlooked, but incredibly valuable, step is getting to know your local fire station, especially when you first move into a new neighborhood.

Firefighters and emergency responders want to know the people in their community. Introducing yourself isn't just a friendly gesture—it helps them put a face to your home, and it gives them valuable context in case you ever need help. When they're familiar with you and your home's layout, they can better keep an eye out and respond quickly if an emergency arises.

Many fire departments across the country also offer community safety programs like Remembering When™, a national initiative from the National Fire Protection Association (NFPA) focused on reducing falls and fire risks among older adults. These programs often offer free home safety checks, educational workshops, and personalized fall prevention tips, sometimes even in partnership with occupational therapists or public health teams.

Firefighters are trained to look for common hazards both inside and outside the home, and they can be excellent allies in creating a safer environment. If you're interested, reach out to your local fire station and ask if they offer home safety visits or participate in Remembering When™. You can also check out the NFPA's resources to see if your community is part of their outreach.

Building these community connections isn't just about safety—it's about creating a support network that's ready to step in when you need it most.

Front Door

OK, let's start right here, right at your front door. This is your first line of defense when it comes to safety and independence, and it's one of the most overlooked parts of the house when we talk about aging in place.

By the time I have walked up to the front door, I've already processed several critical details. Is it a covered space so that I could be out of the rain and not rushing to get the door open? Is there a bench or place where I could put the things in my hands down to get the keys out of my purse and open the front door?

Hazards rarely show up on sunny days when you're well-rested and hands-free. They tend to reveal themselves when it's pouring rain, your arms are full, and you're frazzled, running late, and rushing.

C6 | Home Modification

What I'm Looking For

- **Trip hazards** like uneven concrete, loose bricks, or tight 90-degree turns
- **Step height and depth**: Are the risers too tall? Are the treads deep enough?
- **Grab points**: Is there a handrail? Is there anything sturdy to stabilize yourself?
- **Lighting**: Can you see the path clearly at night? Is the light motion-sensor activated?
- **Thresholds**: Is there a lip to step over at the door itself?
- **Package Shelf**: Is there a place to put things down easily?
- **Multiple doors**: Do I have to manage two doors and a walker to enter the house?

Quick DIY Wins

- ☐ **Repair sidewalk cracks**: This might be as simple as a leveling compound or patch filler for small dips.
- ☐ **Add motion sensor lighting**: You can get a wireless, solar-powered motion light (like the *LEONLITE* or *Ring* smart floodlights) and install it in under 30 minutes.
- ☐ **Use non-slip adhesive strips or paint on steps:** *3M Safety Walk* treads or outdoor textured paint improve traction.
- ☐ **Remove the storm door**: Decrease the fall risk associated with juggling 2 doors, managing a walker and anything else in your hands. Alternative: keep it propped open at all times.
- ☐ **Install a shelf or bench**: Put a small drop-zone shelf by the door so you can set bags down and free your hands to open the door safely.
- ☐ **Contrasting Doormat:** Choose a high-contrast, non-slip mat like the *Notrax Guzzler* in a color that clearly stands out from your flooring.

Age in Place or Find a New Space

Pro Tip: If your floor is dark, avoid using a black mat, as it can visually disappear for someone with low vision. For individuals with dementia, it may even be perceived as a hole in the floor.

When to Call a Pro

- √ **Handrails**: If you have 2–3 steps or more, I always recommend a handrail on both sides. A contractor can install these in wood or aluminum.
    - o For something quick and budget-friendly, look at *Vevor Outdoor Handrails* on Amazon—pre-assembled, durable, and weather-resistant
    - o If you want something higher-end or with more aesthetic flexibility, *Promenaid* is my go-to brand for horizontal reassurance rails in the home and freestanding handrails outside.
- √ **Threshold ramps**: If you're using a walker or wheelchair or just have trouble with that final inch into the doorway, consider a threshold ramp like *EZ-Access Transitions Angled Entry Plate*. It can be installed in minutes and makes a huge difference.

Pro Tip: You can also install a grab bar next to the door frame to have added support.

- √ **Ramped entry:** Install a gently sloped ramped entry (1:12 pitch recommended) with handrails for either the front door or garage.
- √ **Innovative Vertical Platform Lift (VPL):** If you want the look of stairs but the function of a VPL, *FlexStep by LiftUp* saves space and avoids a visible ramp in the front of the house.

Homeowner/Caregiver Self-Audit

- o Is the walking path to the door at least 36" wide?
- o Are steps marked with visible edge contrast?
- o Is there a handrail on both sides of the steps?

C6 | Home Modification

- o Do I have enough light at night to see where I'm walking?
- o Can I open the door and stabilize myself at the same time?
- o Is the threshold flush or ramped?

#OTBrain Insight

Consider your future self. You may not use a cane or walker now, but imagine if you sprained your ankle or had knee surgery—could you still get into your own house without help? That's why even small upgrades like grab bars or wider paths are worth it today.

•••

The Power of Door Automation

Navigating a front door with a walker or wheelchair can feel like an obstacle course. You have to juggle opening the door, steering your mobility aid, and often walking backwards just to get through safely.

It's not just inconvenient, it's a fall waiting to happen. This is where automatic door systems can make a huge difference. Integrated systems like Open Sesame and *AutoSlide* offer hands-free solutions that allow you to control both front doors and interior doors using your voice, a push button, or even an app on your phone.

More affordable, battery-powered systems like *U-Controll* can also be useful, but they come with the hassle of needing regular charging and cannot lock the door, as they work by blocking the strike plate. These options are better suited for interior spaces.

These systems can allow you to unlock your front door, open it, go through, and have it automatically close and lock behind you—all without needing to touch the door. That's a game-changer for less mobile adults and people with spinal cord injuries, allowing them to manage their environments independently.

With smart home integration, you can even pair these systems with Alexa or Siri to control your doors from bed or check who's at the door using a Ring camera. The beauty of these systems is how they let you stay in control of your home. You can coordinate a home appliance delivery and open your garage door remotely to make sure it's placed safely inside the house. This eliminates the risk of falls while trying to answer the door in time.

AutoSlide even offers options to help your pets, like motion sensors or pet tags, so your dog can safely let themselves in and out of the house. At the end of the day, automation isn't just about technology—it's about giving you more freedom, more safety, and more ways to live comfortably on your own terms.

Garage

Let's take a walk through the garage next. Most people think of this as a place to park the car or store seasonal stuff, but for a lot of people, this is the door they use every day. That means we have to treat it with the same respect and scrutiny we give to your front entryway.

I can't tell you how many times I've seen someone using the edge of a workbench or a laundry shelf to push themselves up a step.

Once, it was a step ladder propped up next to concrete steps—with a towel on it. That homeowner needed support to manage the two steep steps down to be able to do his laundry in the garage, "and the metal gets cold, so I figured I'd put a towel on it."

People are clever and adaptive, but these "workarounds" are also clear signs that the environment isn't working for them anymore. He

C6 | Home Modification

didn't consider the fact that if the towel moved, he would also move with it.

Garages are often cluttered, dimly lit, and overlooked in the aging-in-place conversation. But it's an ideal location for a hidden ramp that doesn't advertise that older people with mobility issues may be residing in this space. Garages provide a covered, weather-protected space where you can pull in and take your time exiting the vehicle. Rushing is a major fall risk and one of the most common causes of injury.

What I'm Looking For

- Steps or changes in elevation between the garage and house without a handrail.
- Poor lighting—especially if it's only one overhead bulb or no light at all.
- Clutter near the walking path, especially around doorways.
- Use of furniture, ladders, or shelving as handholds.
- Narrow or uneven pathways that are hard to navigate with bags, carts, or mobility devices.

Quick DIY Wins

- ☐ **Define the edge of steps and thresholds**: Use brightly colored paint or grip strips to visually mark stair edges. This increases contrast and makes each step easier to see.
- ☐ **Add motion-activated lighting:** Something like the *Mr. Beams Battery LED Motion Sensor Light* or *Ring Smart Floodlight* can drastically improve visibility with zero wiring.
- ☐ **Declutter the pathway:** Keep the area from your car to your house clear of bins, shoes, tools, and anything else that could trip you up.

Age in Place or Find a New Space

When to Call a Pro

- √ **Handrails**: If you have even a single step, I recommend a secure hand hold on both sides of the door to have support when going up and going down.
    - o For multiple steps, *Promenaid* is a great option
    - o For space saving, a fold down grab bar from *HealthCraft* is a quality option.
    - o For added grip, *Ponte Giulio* vinyl coated bars stand the test of time
- √ **Floor leveling or threshold ramps**: If it's only a small threshold, Amazon sells everything from 3" rubber scooter ramps to ½" rubber thresholds to minimize the risk of catching a toe.
- √ **Electrical upgrades**: Wireless lights require maintenance with battery changes or charging. If you want lights that are hardwired, automated, or tied to your home assistant, that's a job for a licensed electrician.

Homeowner/Caregiver Self-Audit

- o Is there a sturdy handrail leading from the garage into the house?
- o Is the space well-lit day and night, especially if laundry is in the garage?
- o Can I carry items while keeping one hand free for balance?
- o Am I using ladders, shelving, or furniture for support (red flag)?
- o Is the path from my car to the house clear and unobstructed?
- o Do I have a flush threshold or ramp if needed?

#OTBrain Insight

You want your garage entry to be a safe, secondary path for both day-to-day access and for emergency egress. Make sure the lighting is just as good as in the home, that you have something solid to hold onto to make that transition into the home, and define the path of travel to ensure you keep it clear of trip hazards. Moments of stress and panic can lead to

C6 | Home Modification

unexpected occurrences that increase the risk of falls. Do whatever you can to minimize the risks now.

Laundry Room

Now we're in the laundry room—a space with hidden risks like slippery floors from water or detergent spills. I pay close attention here because laundry often involves repetitive motion, bending, and lifting.

This space may seem simple, but heavy baskets, low machines, and slippery floors are common culprits of injury when people try to do laundry without a proper setup. A solution as simple as having a chair to sit on while folding or transferring clothes can help with fatigue and prevent a loss of balance.

What I'm Looking For

- **Washer/dryer height:** Are they stacked, low to the ground, or front-load vs. top-load?
- **Flooring:** What color is the floor? If detergent spills or water is leaking, is it obvious?
- **Reach zones:** Are detergents and supplies stored in safe, accessible places?
- **Seating:** Is there a stool or chair for seated tasks or to take a break?
- **Lighting:** Can you see clearly when working in this space?
- **Clutter:** Is there space on top of the dryer to put wet laundry before going into the dryer?
- **Clear Space:** Is there enough space to move clothes from one machine to another without twisting or bending dangerously?

Age in Place or Find a New Space

Quick DIY Wins

- ☐ Add a non-slip floor mat or rubber-backed runner (look for beveled edges to prevent tripping).
- ☐ Use sliding storage drawers or laundry pedestals to raise front-load machines.
- ☐ Store detergents and cleaners on waist-height shelves or in open bins for easy grabbing.
- ☐ Add a folding stool or tall chair to use when transferring or folding laundry (*Adjustable Kitchen Perch Stool* is great for this).
- ☐ Install motion sensor or LED lighting strips to brighten a dim laundry nook.
- ☐ Use rolling laundry carts to avoid carrying heavy baskets.
- ☐ In a stackable setup, a motorized chair—like the VELA Independence—can help a person reach the upper dryer while remaining safely seated.

When to Call a Pro

- √ Install pedestal drawers or raise machines for better body mechanics.
- √ Upgrade flooring to something slip-resistant, especially if water often drips from wet clothing. *Altro Illustra* is a good option for this space.
- √ Reconfigure layout: If washer/dryer are hard to access or dangerously tight, a contractor can sometimes flip door hinges or reposition appliances.

Homeowner/Caregiver Self-Audit

- o Can I safely transfer clothes from the washer to the dryer without bending too far or twisting?
- o Is the floor non-slip, even when wet?

C6 | Home Modification

- o Are detergents stored at an easy-to-reach height?
- o Can I sit while doing laundry tasks if I get tired?
- o Is there enough light in the laundry space to work safely?
- o Am I lifting or carrying laundry in a way that strains my back or shoulders?

#OTBrain Insight

Laundry can be repetitive and physical, but it doesn't have to wear you down. A few small changes can turn this necessary activity into a manageable task that fits your body, your energy, and your lifestyle.

Hallway

OK, now we're walking through the hallway, and I'm paying attention to everything from your flooring to shadows on the floor. This is a deceptively simple space, but long, narrow spaces can make vestibular issues worse with no place to sit down if you're dizzy.

Hallways are transition zones, which means people don't think much about paying attention to them. But I've seen more hallway-related falls than I care to count, especially when someone was trying to get to the bathroom urgently.

In the rush, they may not notice that the runner has moved or fail to see an unexpected obstacle because the lighting is too dim. Worse yet, if there's nothing sturdy to grab when balance is momentarily lost, the experience can lead to a lasting fear of falling in that area.

Age in Place or Find a New Space

What I'm Looking For

- At least 36" wide space for walkers and wheelchairs (48" would be even better).
- Lighting—are there burned-out bulbs or not enough light fixtures?
- Clutter, boxes, or decorative furniture that narrows the walking path.
- Touch supports—what is being used for support right now?
- Curling of runner corners, which could be from repeatedly being caught on a walker.
- Loose rugs that move or multiple runners in a row, causing gaps between.

Pro Tip: I especially dislike floor runners that interfere with a clear bedroom to bathroom path of travel for middle-of-the-night trips when someone is half-asleep.

Quick DIY Wins

- ☐ **Remove or secure rugs:** If you're not ready to give up your runner, secure it fully with double-sided rug tape that you can buy easily on *Amazon*.
- ☐ **Add visual contrast:** Use painter's tape or bright duct tape to define step edges or flooring transitions.
- ☐ **Declutter:** Shoes, pet bowls, or decorative benches may look great, but can be dangerous if they narrow the hallway or become trip hazards.
- ☐ **Plug-in motion-sensor nightlights:** *GE LED Motion Lights* or *Vont Lyra* to light the baseboard path at night without waking up the whole house
- ☐ **Plug in LED strips:** *Amazon* sells motion-activated LED lights for under the bed.

C6 | Home Modification

- ☐ **Built-in motion-sensor nightlights:** *SnapPower* is an outlet cover with a built-in nightlight that allows both plugs to remain usable.

Pro Tip: Integrated lights will prevent clients with dementia from unplugging traditional nightlights, thinking they need to be turned off.

When to Call a Pro

- √ **Lighting changes:** Hire a licensed electrician to hard-wire longer motion-activated LED strips along hallway walls to make it light up like the emergency aisle in an airplane. These can be integrated into a smart home system to turn on automatically each evening or respond to voice commands.
- √ **Reassurance rails**: Long hallways can bring on vertigo in some people and in people with Parkinson's, can be a trigger for freezing. *Promenaid* horizontal handrails are a great two-in-one option as they can also be installed with light.

Homeowner/Caregiver Self-Audit

- o Is the hallway at least 36" wide to accommodate mobility aids?
- o Are there any unsecured rugs or runners?
- o Is lighting adequate, especially at night?
- o Is there something to touch or hold while walking through?
- o Are shoes, baskets, or furniture creating trip hazards?
- o Could I navigate the hallway safely if I were dizzy, tired, or using a walker?

#OTBrain Insight

The hallway connects you to the frequently used spaces in your home. When you add light, reduce clutter, and install beautiful reassurance rails that blend in with the environment, it becomes both safe and functional.

Age in Place or Find a New Space

The Story Behind Reassurance Rails

In 2020, Evolving Homes® introduced a new term: *reassurance rails*. It wasn't just a rebrand to move past the stigma of grab bars—it was a complete reframe of how we think about safety, dignity, and design.

The idea came from a simple yet powerful observation: people weren't resisting safety features; they were resisting the language and imagery that accompanied them. The phrase "grab bar" evoked a sense of decline, emergency, or clinical spaces—images that clashed sharply with the sense of pride and emotional connection people felt about their homes.

As an occupational therapist, I found that the people who most needed support were often the most reluctant to accept it. But in deeper conversations, a new truth emerged. Clients, especially proactive ones, weren't rejecting support entirely. They just couldn't see themselves needing to "grab" anything. The word alone felt like a surrender. Others admitted that while they sometimes felt unsteady, their need was intermittent. They wanted something subtler. Something they could engage with on their terms, not a fixture that shouted "frailty."

That's when I started to think about the idea of grab bars providing light reassurance. Instead of isolated vertical bars next to a toilet or inside a shower stall, I proposed a continuous horizontal path of support, usually from the bedroom to the bathroom, down long hallways, around corners and from front door to car.

These rails offered a comforting, tactile presence—a gentle guide, not a lifeline. Simply running a hand along the wall-mounted support gave clients the reassurance that if they did lose their balance, help was quite literally within reach. And because the rails were securely mounted into the studs, clients had a high level of trust in their safety and reliability.

When I introduced this idea to designers, architects, and contractors, something clicked. The terminology, the intent, and the design possibilities opened doors, quite literally and figuratively. Reassurance rails became an accessible concept, both linguistically and emotionally. Since then, many professionals have shared with me how easily clients accepted these installations when framed in this way.

C6 | Home Modification

When Safety Looks Like Design

For some of my patients with Parkinson's disease, I've noticed a specific hallway hazard—corners. Many people with Parkinson's experience neck stiffness and don't turn segmentally, which means they often misjudge the depth of a hallway corner and bump into it while turning.

A common solution is to place a strip of brightly colored duct tape along the edge to provide a visual cue and help with environmental scanning. It works, but let's be honest, it's not pretty. I've also seen clear plastic bumpers used to protect the wall, but to me, those feel more like commercial building fixes than something that belongs in a warm, inviting home.

One of my favorite #OTBrain design moments came from solving this problem in a way that felt more human and less like a workaround.

I discovered that using intentional color contrast with paint wasn't just effective, it was beautiful. By simply painting one wall a different color from the other, I created a strong visual cue that naturally drew the eye and helped guide my patient to make that 90-degree turn safely. The best part? It didn't look like a safety feature at all. It looked like thoughtful design—an accent wall anyone might choose.

These are the solutions I love: the ones that don't rely on ugly tape, baby-proofing gadgets, or institutional fixes. Solutions that are smart, subtle, and honor both the person and the home they love. That's #OTBrain at its best.

Age in Place or Find a New Space

Living Room

Now we're in the living room—usually one of the coziest, most relaxing spaces in the house. When I walk into this room, I'm looking for trip hazards like rugs in the path of travel, soft or too low furniture that's hard to get out of, and dangerous glass coffee tables with sharp edges.

This is the space where we gather, nap, watch TV, or host friends. But it's also one of the most common places where people fall. The instinct is often to immediately remove all rugs to eliminate trip hazards, but I like to take a step back and start by asking: Why is this rug important to you? It might be sentimental. It might provide warmth. Or it might be the bright, energizing color that makes the space feel alive. The key is to ask more questions and truly understand the homeowner's priorities before jumping to solutions.

I was in a client's home recently where the coffee table was made of glass—a clear safety risk. The rugs had curling corners, creating trip hazards, and the oversized armchair completely swallowed this tiny woman. Not only did it put her in poor posture, but she also had to use momentum to stand up every single time—a major fall risk.

But here's the thing. She had plenty of good reasons for what, on the surface, seemed like a trainwreck of a space. The solution isn't always to strip the room down to nothing. It's about understanding why something matters to the person and finding safer ways to keep the things they love.

What I'm Looking For

> **Seating height, depth, and firmness**: Can you get up and down without assistance? Is your back supported when you are sitting as far back as you can?

C6 | Home Modification

- **Furniture layout**: Is there enough space to maneuver safely, especially with mobility aids?
- **Coffee tables and ottomans:** Are corners rounded? Can they be moved easily if needed? Is there color contrast to the floor so the edges are defined? Could a soft ottoman work instead?
- **Rugs:** Are they secured, low-profile, and high-contrast?
- **Lighting:** Can someone safely navigate the space at night?
- **Electrical cords:** Are they tucked away from walking paths?
- **TV or remote clutter:** Are they easily accessible without bending or straining?

Quick DIY Wins

- ☐ Remove or secure area rugs with double-sided carpet tape or rug grippers.
- ☐ Use painter's tape to outline the edges of glass tables temporarily while you look for replacements with better visibility
- ☐ Add plug-in motion-activated lighting near outlets or floor level (*GE Motion Sensor Night Lights* work well)
- ☐ Clear out clutter like magazine piles, extension cords, or low baskets in walk paths.
- ☐ To control your lights without the complexity of a full smart home setup, consider an innovative solution: the *Lotus Ring and Switch Cover System*—a simple, non-WiFi alternative that offers effortless convenience.

When to Call a Pro

- √ **Furniture replacement:** If low or unstable chairs are a problem, consider replacing them with investment-quality, firm-seat options like *Golden Technologies* lift chairs or chairs with 20–21" seat heights.

Age in Place or Find a New Space

- √ **Lighting upgrades:** Have an electrician install wall sconces or ceiling lighting if the space is dark and full of glare.
- √ **Flooring changes:** Replace slippery laminate or plush carpet with low-pile, slip-resistant flooring for better stability. Good quality LVP has a soft buffer to absorb sound and some impact (without allowing too much movement between boards as with lower quality ones.)
- √ **Home automation:** Use smart voice assistants to simplify TV and lighting controls.

Homeowner/Caregiver Self-Audit

- o Can I sit down and stand up from all the chairs without struggling?
- o Is there at least 36" of clearance between major furniture pieces?
- o Are there any glass, sharp-edged, or low tables in the way?
- o Are rugs secured or removed entirely?
- o Do I have enough light to safely navigate the room at night?
- o Are there cords, baskets, or other obstacles in my walking path?

#OTBrain Insight

The living room should support your occupation of watching TV or chatting with friends and not promote prolonged poor posture. Choose comfort that respects your mobility, not just your style.

··

Furniture Selection

All the planning in the world for structural and electrical won't matter if your furniture choices don't support accessibility. I see it all the time—people pick furniture based on looks alone. But function matters just as much as form.

C6 | Home Modification

Flow and Navigation

When you're thinking about furniture, don't just think about the pieces—think about the layout and how you move through the space. Are you making sharp turns around recliners or dodging oversized coffee tables? Your layout should make movement easy and safe, especially if you're using a walker, a cane, or just trying to carry a cup of coffee from the kitchen to the living room without a spill.

The ideal setup is a clear, direct path of travel from the kitchen to the living room—one that isn't chopped up by rugs, carpet edges, or wandering ottomans. A little planning here can make everyday life so much smoother.

Sofas

The most common problems I see with sofas are that they're either too low to get out of easily or too deep to support good posture. So, what's the best seat height to look for? Most people feel comfortable with a seat height between 18 and 20 inches, where the hips sit slightly above the knees to make standing up easier. But here's my simple rule of thumb: look for a seat that's about two inches above your knee, so that when you sit down, your hips are higher than your knees. This makes it easier to get up.

Body size matters—a petite person's femur is much shorter than a towering person six feet tall. Deep couches can force shorter users into a rounded-back posture, which puts strain on both the joints and the muscles. Deep seats also require more effort to scoot forward to the edge before standing—a common challenge and a safety risk. Right-sizing your furniture makes sure that everyone in your home can sit comfortably and, most importantly, stand up independently.

And let's talk about foam quality—it really does matter. Inexpensive foam breaks down fast, which makes getting up harder over time and increases the risk of falls. For anyone using a wheelchair or recovering from illness, transferring to a surface that's too soft—like memory foam—is actually pretty dangerous. That super cushy couch might look cozy, but if it sinks a couple of inches when you sit down, it's going to be tough to get back up, and even harder to do a slide board transfer safely.

Chairs

One of the most common problems I see with living room chairs is the bucket seat style, where the knees sit higher than the hips. This design forces people to scoot "uphill" to reach the edge of the seat, making it much harder to stand, especially since these chairs are often lower to the ground. They frequently come with a matching ottoman, which adds another layer of risk. Ottomans are a very common trip hazard, particularly for people with decreased neck mobility from cervical surgeries or for individuals with Parkinson's, who may not always remember to look down due to neck stiffness.

If the goal is to comfortably put your feet up and rest, I usually recommend investing in a good quality lift chair, like those from *Golden Technologies*. These chairs support safe, assisted sit-to-stand transfers and can also recline completely flat for a mid-day nap. Some models even include a "twilight" feature that elevates the legs above the heart—an excellent option for encouraging ankle swelling to shift toward the bladder when used about two hours before bedtime. This can help reduce swelling and may even decrease the number of nighttime bathroom trips.

Lift chairs can be expensive, and preferences really vary. I've had clients who were happy to invest $4,000 in a top-quality chair with a 20-year guarantee, while others preferred to buy a brand-new $400 lift chair every year instead. Both followed the path that made the most sense for them. In my opinion, as long as the chair is safe, sturdy, and in good condition, it's the right answer for that person. There's no one-size-fits-all solution—it's about what works best for their life and comfort.

What to Look For

> **Seat heights** that make standing easier.
> **Quality foam** for long-term comfort.
> **Materials** that can withstand moisture.
> **Color contrast** between the sofa edge and the flooring below.

Rug Safety

I understand the reasons why people resist getting rid of rugs. They add warmth, color, and a cozy feel to a room. But it's also true that rugs can also be one of the most common trip hazards if we're not careful. The key is to choose them wisely and set them up with safety in mind.

Low-pile or flat-weave rugs are your best bet. They're easier to walk over, especially if you're using a walker or cane, and they won't catch your toe the way thicker, plush rugs can. Tassels might look charming, but they're a tripping risk—trimming them down or avoiding them altogether is a smart move.

I always recommend making sure there's a strong color contrast between your rug and the floor underneath. It's a small detail that makes a big difference for people with low vision or those who don't always remember to look down. And don't forget to secure the edges with double-sided carpet tape or a non-slip rug pad to keep everything firmly in place—no sliding, no curling, no surprises.

Color Contrast, Texture, and Fabric Choices

When selecting furniture, upholstery isn't just about style. It's about making life easier. If incontinence, spills, or heavy use is on your radar, look for urethane-coated fabrics.

They're super easy to clean and offer excellent stain resistance—perfect for homes with grandkids, pets, or just everyday life. No need for awkward conversations ☺ Just smart, thoughtful planning.

Age in Place or Find a New Space

And here's where color and texture really matter. Color isn't just a design choice, it's functional. Strong contrasts between walls, floors, and furniture help people with low vision or cognitive changes navigate more safely. Avoid all-white bathrooms or monochromatic spaces that can hide depth changes, edges, or steps. When you're picking out your couch and flooring, try to coordinate both at the same time to ensure a clear color contrast. This helps prevent someone from misjudging the distance and missing the seat entirely.

If colors are similar, adding texture is another powerful strategy. Texture gives your brain more information. Using textured upholstery or accent elements can help people better distinguish surfaces and move more confidently through a room.

Pro Tip: Encourage people to back up until they can feel the couch fabric behind their knees, then reach back for the sofa arms, before gently lowering themselves down. This is a small habit that can make a big difference in preventing falls.

Design Traps to Avoid

There are a few common design choices that look great on paper but can quietly create safety risks in real life.

One of the biggest culprits? Glass tables. They're beautiful, but they're hard to see, especially in low light, and it's easy to misjudge where the edge is when placing food or scooting in to sit on the couch. I always prefer sturdy wooden tables that have a strong color contrast against the floor so you can clearly see where they are. Another great option is a soft ottoman with a tray on top. It's stable, practical, and easy to move if you need more space.

Sharp corners are another thing to watch out for. They can cause nasty skin tears or painful bruises if you catch your hip or leg on the edge. I recommend rectangular tables with rounded corners instead. (Round

C6 | Home Modification

tables can tip over pretty easily if someone leans on them for support, so rectangular with rounded edges is usually the safest bet.)

And let's talk about slippery surfaces. Marble might look luxurious, but it's not your friend when it comes to fall prevention. If you already have slippery floors, you can make them safer by adding large, secured area rugs with grip tape or by considering injury-prevention flooring options. A safe home doesn't mean you have to sacrifice style. It just means choosing features that work with you, not against you.

Kitchen

Let's move into the kitchen—the hub of daily activity. Whether you love cooking, meal prepping, or just reheating leftovers, this space gets used constantly. And it's full of hidden risks most people never think about until something goes wrong.

The kitchen is one of the most demanding rooms in the house, both cognitively and physically. You're managing heat, sharp objects, multitasking, and often working in tight quarters.

When I assess a kitchen, my goal is to ensure everything is within reach, reduce the need to twist or bend, and lower the risk of injuries from falls, burns, or even a sudden urge to bake or deep-clean.

I've had clients slip off step ladders while reaching for rarely used items on high shelves, and others who were inspired to clean under the sink, only to find they couldn't get back up again.

What I'm Looking For

- **Appliance placement:** Can you use the oven, microwave, and dishwasher without bending or reaching too far?

Age in Place or Find a New Space

- **Storage access:** Are commonly used items within easy reach, between knee and shoulder height?
- **Lighting:** Is the workspace bright and free from glare and shadows? Is there both overhead lighting and task lighting? Are there lights in the cabinets?
- **Stove safety:** Are controls on the front or back? Is there a risk of fire?
- **Flooring:** Is it non-slip and easy to clean? Is it a matte finish to reduce glare?
- **Seating:** Is there a place to sit while doing prep work if needed?
- **Path width:** Is there at least 36" of clearance to maneuver safely?
- **Countertop:** Is the counter clear of clutter? Can you use the counter to slide heavy pots instead of lifting them? Is it free from glare?
- **Cabinet style:** Do you need to keep your head upside down to see inside lower cabinets?

Quick DIY Wins

- ☐ Move heavy, frequently used items (like pots or blenders) to waist-height cabinets.
- ☐ Install pull-down cabinet shelves or use lazy Susans to avoid reaching into deep spaces (brands like *Rev-A-Shelf* are easy to install).
- ☐ Add under-cabinet lighting for better visibility—battery-powered LED strips also work great.
- ☐ Add a rolling prep stool or seat for cooking tasks (*Drive Medical Kitchen Stool* is adjustable and stable)
- ☐ Keep frequently used items in the same location to reduce mental and physical strain
- ☐ Consider easy to install fire safety technologies if memory or attention is a concern. *Ome Kitchen* is a smart stove knob that can be controlled via app. *iGuard* is a smart shutoff device. Cooktop Safety has boil over prediction. So many different ways to approach the problem!

C6 | Home Modification

When to Call a Pro

- √ **Install layered lighting:** If a workspace is too dark, consider having an electrician put in ambient, task, and accent lighting. If there is space, install cabinet lighting for ease of use.
- √ **Smart Home Integration:** It can be difficult to get all the apps to play nicely together, so having an integrator come to set up voice-activated lights, blinds, smart faucets, and app-controlled microwaves may be worth your time and money.
- √ **Appliance upgrades:** Install a wall oven or raised dishwasher to eliminate bending. Install an under-counter microwave to avoid reaching over a hot stove. For a stove, look for easy to read appliance controls. Front knobs are easier to access and safer than reaching over a hot stove to adjust temperatures. Induction hotplates are ideal to decrease the risk of burns and are preferred for fire safety in congregate living. For a fridge, consider styles that offer flexibility to move a freezer compartment to a fridge so that both compartments could be accessed at wheelchair level if needed.
- √ **Flooring replacement:** If the surface is slick or hard on joints, upgrade to cushioned vinyl or slip-resistant tile like *Altro* or *Tarkett*.
- √ **Invest in a motorized chair**, such as the *VELA Independence*, to perform household tasks while seated—helping to conserve energy and reduce the fear of falling.

Homeowner/Caregiver Self-Audit

- o Can I reach the microwave, stove, and fridge without overreaching or bending too far?
- o Are my most-used items stored at easy-to-reach heights (not on top shelves or deep drawers)?
- o Is the stove safe—are knobs clearly visible and within reach?
- o Can I sit comfortably to prep food if needed?

Age in Place or Find a New Space

- o Are the floors slip-resistant and easy to navigate with a cane or walker?
- o Is the lighting bright and evenly spread across work surfaces?

#OTBrain Insight
The kitchen can become a space that supports your health, safety, and independence with little changes. Don't wait until things get hard to do something about it. Start early so you can keep doing what you love.

Flexible and Accessible Kitchen Solutions

For kitchens that are shared by people of different heights or for those who need to work while seated, adjustable-height countertops can be a fantastic option. Brands like *Granberg, Ropox*, and *Pressalit* offer counters that can move up or down to match the user's needs.

This is especially helpful for wheelchair users, people who are easily fatigued, or anyone who wants to work in a seated position. These counters can even be configured to include an induction stove or sink, creating a fully functional, adaptable workspace.

Pro Tip: I like to install a height-adjustable countertop early on so it can be used right away by all family members for joint protection and comfort. If maximizing storage space is the priority and there's no immediate need for height adjustability, I often recommend having a woodworker build a matching cabinet on wheels. This cabinet can be stored under the sink until knee clearance is needed. When that time comes, the rolling cabinet can easily be moved—either temporarily or permanently—to create the necessary space.

Adjustable-height upper cabinets are another great solution when storage is hard to reach. Many of the same brands make motorized cabinets where the inside shelves can lower to the countertop, or the entire cabinet can slide down and out toward you. This removes the need for

C6 | Home Modification

step stools and dramatically reduces the risk of falls, especially when working from a seated position.

For lower storage, pull-out shelves are a game-changer. Retrofitting existing tower or base cabinets with fully extendable pull-out shelves—like those from *ShelfGenie*—makes access much easier and reduces the need to reach, bend, or dig for items in the back. I often recommend replacing traditional base cabinets with large drawer-style units instead.

Drawer-style storage offers much better visibility and allows you to pull items directly toward you, eliminating the need to crouch or bend over. I prefer U-shaped or H-shaped drawer pulls, which can be opened with the side of your hand—or even a foot—rather than requiring a tripod grip. *IKEA* offers great, budget-friendly options with customizable organization systems that work well for this.

When you start combining these smart, flexible storage solutions, you create a kitchen that moves with you, adapts to your needs, and helps you work more safely and efficiently. Whether you're standing, sitting, or working alongside others, these upgrades make everyday tasks feel easier and more comfortable.

Home Office

Let's step into the home office or whatever space is being used for bills, planning, or computer work. This room might not seem risky at first glance, but it's often where I see a mix of physical strain and cognitive clutter that can impact function and independence.

For many people, the "office" is a catchall zone—a desk, some files, a laptop, maybe a printer. But this space often becomes a quiet source of stress from sitting in dining chairs for hours at a time with cords

Age in Place or Find a New Space

running in every direction and piles of papers that make it hard to find important documents in a crisis or create a fall hazard if they spill to the floor.

This room is just as important as the kitchen or bathroom because this is where important Instrumental Activities of Daily Living (IADL) skills like managing money, scheduling appointments, and organizing important documents occur. Whether someone is still working, managing a household, or communicating with healthcare providers, the environment needs to support them organizationally and ergonomically, not make things harder.

What I'm Looking For

> - **Seating:** Is the chair supportive? Does it have arms and an appropriate height?
> - **Lighting:** Is it bright enough to prevent eye strain and fatigue?
> - **Desk setup:** Is the monitor at eye level? Is there space for writing or reading?
> - **Clutter:** Are cords, papers, and supplies organized or creating stress and tripping hazards?
> - **Accessibility:** Are essential documents (medical records, emergency contacts, medication lists) easy to find?
> - **Tech overload:** Are there too many small devices or confusing gadgets?

Quick DIY Wins

- ☐ Sort and store important documents in a labeled binder or folder—emergency info should be ready to grab and go in case of an unexpected need for hospitalization.
- ☐ Low-cost ergonomics: Use desk risers or a stack of books to raise screens to eye level.

C6 | Home Modification

- ☐ Add task lighting with a gooseneck LED desk lamp (adjustable brightness helps with vision changes).
- ☐ Use cord organizers or cable sleeves to eliminate tripping and tangling hazards.
- ☐ For easy access - Make sure to keep medications list updated for emergency personnel.
- ☐ Replace an old chair with one that has armrests and adjustable height (*Modway* and *Staples Hyken* are affordable and supportive options).
- ☐ Install voice assistants (like Alexa or Google Nest) to simplify reminders, lists, and calls.
- ☐ Invest in an adjustable desk (like IKEA's sit-to-stand) to accommodate different body sizes and provide optimal working heights, including for wheelchair users.

When to Call a Pro

- √ **Decluttering help**: A professional organizer can create customized storage systems that improve access.
- √ **Streamline technology**: A smart home integrator can help to eliminate duplication and clutter.
- √ **Lighting upgrades**: If natural light is limited, have an electrician install brighter overhead lights or install wall-mounted fixtures.

Homeowner/Caregiver Self-Audit

- o Is the chair supportive, with a seat height that allows both feet to touch the floor?
- o Can I sit at the desk for more than 10–15 minutes without back or neck pain?
- o Is the lighting bright and well-positioned for reading or computer use?

Age in Place or Find a New Space

- o Are cords out of the way and secured?
- o Can I quickly find emergency contact information or health documents if needed?
- o Is the space free of clutter that makes it mentally or physically hard to function?

#OTBrain Insight

A well-organized office is the environment that best supports the occupation of running your household. When your desk is organized, your thinking often is, too. Being able to find important documents easily is one of the greatest gifts we can give ourselves as we age in place.

Flooring Matters: The Memory Foam Mistake

It's easy to think that soft flooring—like memory foam carpet padding—is the perfect choice, especially for people who are afraid of falling. I actually have memory foam carpet in my own house because when I was shopping, the carpet salesman told me it would extend the life of the carpet, even though it cost about three times more than standard padding. And for many spaces, it's fine.

But I've learned from experience that memory foam is not ideal for an office. I once worked with a client who was prone to falls and had reasoned that installing memory foam throughout his home would reduce his injury risk. What he discovered instead was that it created new challenges. In his office, his chair would sink into the foam, and after a few minutes, the wheels would get stuck in deep grooves, and it became incredibly hard to roll his chair away from the desk.

His unique set of Parkinson's symptoms included freezing, which made it difficult for him to pick his feet up from the memory foam floor to shift his weight. The memory foam padding actually became more of a trip hazard than a safety net.

C6 | Home Modification

In his case, the solution was to remove the memory foam and install standard carpet padding instead—a much better balance between comfort and the ability to move safely and freely.

When it comes to office spaces, the best flooring is one that's firm, smooth, and allows easy movement of chairs, mobility aids, and feet. Sometimes, what feels safer in theory can actually limit independence in real life.

Guest Bedroom/Exercise Room

Let's walk into the guest bedroom that often doubles as the exercise room. Many people think of this as the least-used room in the house, but actually, it often ends up being the one that matters most in a moment of need. Whether it's an aging parent staying over, a recovering spouse sleeping separately after surgery, or a caregiver needing a comfortable place to rest, this room deserves thoughtful attention.

When assessing a guest bedroom, I consider who is likely to use it and under what circumstances. Will they face mobility challenges? Might they become disoriented at night? If it's being used as an exercise space most of the time, is there enough room to store the equipment away during a family visit without creating a fall hazard?

What I'm Looking For

- **Bed height and firmness:** Can a guest easily get in and out of bed without strain?
- **Pathway:** Is there at least 36" of clear space to move with a walker or cane?

Age in Place or Find a New Space

- ➤ **Lighting:** Is there a lamp that's easy to reach and operate from the bed?
- ➤ **Nightstand access:** Are glasses, medications, and a phone or call button reachable?
- ➤ **Clutter:** Is the room free of storage piles, workout gear, or "temporary" items?
- ➤ **Emergency plan:** If an older guest needed assistance, how would they let you know?

Quick DIY Wins

- ☐ **Raise** bed height with furniture risers (*Amazon*) to get it to above-the-knee level.
- ☐ **Lower** bed height by replacing the 9"box spring with a 2" Bunkie Board available at mattress stores or purchase a platform frame.
- ☐ Add motion-sensor plug-in nightlights along the baseboards (*Vont* or *GE*).
- ☐ Keep a flashlight, water bottle, and a way to get attention on the nightstand like a bell.
- ☐ Install a bed assist bar if your guest has mobility issues (<u>Medline</u> is simple)
- ☐ Pamper a guest with friction-reducing sheets and pajamas to move easily (<u>Comfort Linen</u>).
- ☐ Clear out clutter, cords, or bins that may have crept into the space over time.

When to Call a Pro

- √ Install horizontal reassurance rails to get from bedroom to bathroom easily.
- √ Widen the doorway for accessible use.

C6 | Home Modification

- √ Install an intercom or monitoring device if the guest has medical needs.
- √ Upgrade to a mattress with firm edge support to avoid slipping off a soft bed.
- √ Add smart technology for voice-activated lighting, climate control, or call-for-help features (Alexa, Google Home).

Homeowner/Caregiver Self-Audit

- o Is the bed height appropriate for someone with limited strength or flexibility?
- o Is there clear space to walk around the bed with a walker or cane?
- o Can a guest reach the lamp, phone, and water without leaning or twisting?
- o Is the room truly ready for someone, or is it being used for storage? Clutter is a fall risk.
- o Would a guest feel safe and supported here if they were recovering from illness or surgery?
- o Is there a clear plan for calling for help if needed?

#OTBrain Insight

A guest room isn't just for guests—it's a flexible space that can serve many roles, from separating family members during illness to supporting short- or long-term caregiving needs. When you prepare that room with mobility needs in mind, you send a powerful message: You matter. Your safety and comfort matter. And we want you to feel welcome, so you'll want to come back.

Age in Place or Find a New Space

Designing an Exercise Space

If you're planning to age in place, exercise isn't optional. It has to become a central part of your life. One of the best ways to reinforce this mindset is to dedicate space in your home that's specifically for exercise. I often tell my clients: When you give something enough space in your life, you're showing how important it is to you.

A great example is the guest room. Many people use their guest room only a few times a year, but for the other 90 percent of the time, it just sits there. Why not turn it into a dedicated exercise space when it's not in use? This is far more effective than trying to squeeze in a workout in your office, hoping you won't knock over a stack of papers or trip over cords while following a virtual class.

When I help people design these spaces, the first thing I recommend is installing a cushioned, gym-style floor. This creates a safe area where you can practice one of the most essential skills: getting up and down from the floor. I've seen it over and over. Once people can do this confidently, their fear of falling decreases dramatically. That fear is one of the biggest barriers to staying active, and when you can eliminate it, everything changes.

I also recommend installing a full-length mirror. A lot of people think they're standing up straight, but when I show them a picture or video, they realize they're leaning to one side or carrying their weight unevenly. A mirror gives you real-time feedback so you can immediately correct your posture and prevent long-term imbalances before they lead to falls or injuries. You want to be the one who notices, not your therapist months down the road.

Another great addition is a TV or screen for streaming virtual classes or joining live sessions with friends. There are so many options now with on-demand programs, YouTube exercise routines, and interactive group workouts. The social connection and variety make it easier to stick with your routine. Honestly, there's so much out there now that it's hard to come up with a good excuse not to do it.

C6 | Home Modification

One of my favorite features to add to an at-home exercise space is a horizontal bar installed in front of the mirror. I love using *Promenaid* bars here, the same ones I recommend for reassurance rails. They can be securely anchored to the studs, and they offer a sturdy support for stretching, assisted squats, and balance work. I often have people use the bar to stretch their hamstrings by propping their foot on it or to safely build the quad strength needed for sit-to-stand transfers.

Exercise is a lifelong journey. Designing a space in your home that makes it easy to move, practice, and grow shows your commitment to protecting your independence and keeping your life full of the things that matter most to you. It's one of the smartest investments you can make in your future.

Guest Bathroom

Let's step into the guest bathroom. It might be the smallest room in the house, but it plays a huge role, especially when someone is visiting, recovering, or helping out long-term. This is where thoughtful details can truly shine.

Guest bathrooms are often compact and designed with aesthetics in mind like beautiful tiles, pedestal sinks, and decorative rugs. But when I evaluate them, I'm asking different questions: Can someone safely get in and out of the shower? Is there a place to steady themselves near the toilet? Are the essentials within reach without stretching or bending?

One reason I like to bring this up during a home assessment is that I often get a flurry of questions around the holidays, when people suddenly realize the guest bathroom may not meet their visitors' needs.

I remember a friend telling me about her independent, widowed father who had come to stay over the holidays. Her bathtub was deeper

Age in Place or Find a New Space

than he was used to, and after struggling for nearly an hour to get out, he finally had to call her for help. She felt awful, and he felt embarrassed. My goal is to help you avoid these uncomfortable interactions as much as possible.

What I'm Looking For

- **Shower/tub access:** Is there a step-over edge? Is there a grab bar or seat available?
- **Toilet support:** Is the toilet too low to get up from? Can they reach the toilet paper?
- **Lighting:** Would someone have enough light to see during a nighttime bathroom trip?
- **Storage and reach:** Are towels, toiletries, and supplies within easy reach?
- **Floor safety:** Are rugs secured? Is the surface slick when wet?
- **Emergency backup:** Could a guest call for help from here if needed?

Quick DIY Wins

- ☐ Add a rubber bathmat both inside and outside the tub/shower. I look for commercial kitchen-style ones with holes to catch the water.
- ☐ Use suction-based grab bars as a low-cost, **TEMPORARY** solution and provide clear instructions on how to check their security prior to bathing. ** **VERY IMPORTANT** **
- ☐ Add a raised toilet seat or portable toilet safety frame. 3n1 commodes can also be used.
- ☐ Place motion sensor nightlights in the hallway and bathroom to guide nighttime visits.
- ☐ Keep essentials like towels and toiletries between waist and shoulder height: Use a small shelf or over-the-toilet storage.

C6 | Home Modification

- ☐ If needed, place a rubber-backed bath rug with beveled edges to prevent tripping.

When to Call a Pro

- √ Install permanent grab bars in the shower and near the toilet, anchored into wall studs. Choose beautiful bars that blend seamlessly with the environment and style.
- √ Replace deep tubs with a walk-in shower if the room will be used frequently by someone with mobility concerns.
- √ Replace toilet with a comfort-height model.
- √ Reconfigure tight layouts to allow better movement or space for assistive devices.

Homeowner/Caregiver Self-Audit

- o Is the shower or tub easy to get into without stepping high or twisting?
- o Is there a secure place to hold onto when sitting or standing from the toilet?
- o Is the lighting sufficient, especially for nighttime use?
- o Are there rugs, cords, or clutter that could cause someone to trip?
- o Are towels, soap, and other supplies within easy reach—no bending or tiptoeing required?
- o If someone had a fall here, could they call for help?

#OTBrain Insight

Safety doesn't have to come at the expense of style. The ideal guest bathroom includes grab bars that blend seamlessly into the design—hidden in plain sight—offering both elegance and security.

Age in Place or Find a New Space

Blocking: The Unsung Hero of Home Planning

If there's one thing every project should include, it's blocking. Most people think of it only in terms of hanging cabinets, but its value extends far beyond that, especially when it comes to aging in place.

Blocking is one of the simplest, most cost-effective ways to plan ahead, especially when the walls are already open. In bathrooms, blocking is critical for securely mounting shower seats and grab bars. In bedrooms, it allows for my favorite reassurance rails—horizontal rails that offer peace of mind when moving from bedroom to bathroom.

Even if you're not planning to install these items right away, chances are someone will want them down the line. So, if you're remodeling (not building from scratch), ask your contractor to add extra blocking now while the walls are open. You won't have to hold your breath when it's time to drill. You'll know exactly where support can go, and you'll be confident it's secure.

Pro tip: While the blocking is being installed, take clear photos with a measuring tape in the frame. Save them, digitally or printed, so you (or a future homeowner) can easily reference the location during future installations. It's a small step with a big payoff when the time comes to add grab bars or other supports.

Standard ADA guidelines recommend placing blocking between 33 and 36 inches high. That's a good starting point but I prefer to plan more generously. I usually recommend adding horizontal blocking from knee to shoulder height, and ideally on all walls in key areas. That gives you the flexibility to add support where you need it, without guessing or compromising function. The only exceptions are specific fixtures like fold-down seats or extra-long grab bars that require unique placement points.

If you're too far into a project to add blocking or working under a time crunch—say, preparing for a rehab discharge—prefabricated fiberglass showers with integrated wood backers are a great second-best option. I use them often in fast-paced situations because they're safe, sturdy, and ready to go without the wait.

Blocking may not be glamorous, but it gives you the power to adapt your space to fit your needs, now and in the future. It turns the unknown into something manageable, giving you peace of mind that your home will continue to work for you.

More importantly, planning early means fewer compromises later. Your goal is just to get the space as close as you can to what you think you might need, and because blocking is so much cheaper to put in when the walls are down, it's automatic savings and peace of mind for later.

Why Retrofitting Is Risky

One reason people underestimate the value of blocking is that they've never experienced the headache of retrofitting. On drywall, finding studs is easy. But behind layers of tile and cement board? Not so much. Stud finders usually fail, and you're left guessing.

In some cases, if the tile doesn't extend to the ceiling, you can use the visible studs in the drywall above as a guide—but even that has its risks. Homes are rarely built identically. While 16 inches on center is standard stud spacing, I've seen homes with 12-inch spacing for hurricane resistance or irregular spacing around windows and doors.

And here's the tricky part: Windows in showers often have multiple studs for support, but I've also seen framing where the studs below the window don't align with those above it. That's a real problem if you're relying on upper placement to map out lower support. Once the drill comes out, all fingers are crossed.

If you're dealing with a newly renovated bathroom with fresh tile? It gets even more nerve-wracking. A small misstep in drywall can be patched. Tile—especially glass tile—doesn't offer that same grace. Crack a tile, and you're likely stuck without a replacement match. The risk of damage is high, and the cost of fixing it is even higher.

Age in Place or Find a New Space

Master Bedroom

"We're in the master bedroom now—the place where your day begins and ends. This should be a space that supports rest, ease of movement, and safety."

When I walk into a bedroom, I'm thinking about fatigue at the end of a long day and how that can make it harder for people to get their legs into bed at night. I'm thinking about nighttime bathroom trips and that path of travel to the bathroom. I'm thinking about how someone might wake up stiff, possibly lightheaded, and try to get out of a bed that's too low or too soft.

This is often the first space where I hear, "I'm fine, I've done it this way for years." But I want to know: Could you still do it like that if you were weak from the flu? What if you just had knee surgery or were recovering from a fall? Could you still manage this space safely?

What I'm Looking For

- **Access**: Is it a first-floor bedroom? What is the escape route in case of fire?
- **Clutter:** Are there clothes, shoes, or cords on the floor that could trip someone?
- **Path to the bathroom**: Is it clear, lit, and wide enough for mobility devices?
- **Seating:** Is there a safe spot to sit while dressing or putting on shoes?
- **Lighting:** Can someone light the path to the bathroom without getting out of bed?
- **Voice-controlled options:** Do they have a way to get ready for bed that takes less energy? Automatic Alexa routines like closing blinds, turning off lights, initiating sleep routines, checking the

C6 | Home Modification

security system is engaged, and doors are locked are very useful for bedtime.
- **Nightstand access:** Are water, medications, glasses, and phone within reach?
- **Bed height:** Can the person sit and stand without effort or flopping onto the mattress? Can their feet touch the floor or do they dangle?
- **Bed mobility:** Can they get in and out of the bed easily and safely to use the bathroom?

Quick DIY Wins

- ☐ Declutter, declutter, declutter!
- ☐ Use off-set hinges like *SwingClear* to widen a doorway by 2".
- ☐ Ideally, no rugs in the bedroom (carpet is fine) but if it's a non-negotiable, use non-slip area rugs with beveled edges or secure current rugs with carpet tape.
- ☐ Install motion-activated under-bed LED strip lighting and touch lamps on the nightstand.
- ☐ Keep a small bench or chair with arms for dressing in a seated position.
- ☐ Keep nightstand essentials—like water, phone, glasses, and medications—within easy reach.
- ☐ Place a grabber tool in the nightstand to retrieve items that have fallen without excessive bending. Falls often happen when attempting to retrieve something that has rolled under the bed.

When to Call a Pro

- √ If the mattress is too soft or too firm, consider switching to a medium-firm model that allows easy transfer in and out.
- √ Widen the bedroom-to-bathroom doorway if someone uses a walker or wheelchair.

Age in Place or Find a New Space

- √ Installing reassurance rails along the bed or wall for safe path of travel to bathroom at night (*Promenaid* rails offer sleek, supportive options)
- √ Have an electrician hardwire motion activated lights to light up the path to the bathroom and increase light in the bedroom.

Homeowner/Caregiver Self-Audit

- o Can I sit down on the bed and stand back up easily?
- o Is the path from bed to bathroom clear and wide enough for a walker?
- o Can I reach my nightstand items without twisting or leaning?
- o Is the floor free of shoes, laundry, or tripping hazards?
- o Is there lighting I can operate from the bed, without getting up first?
- o Is there a place to sit safely when dressing?

#OTBrain Insight

Your bedroom is where you're most vulnerable—groggy, tired, sometimes unsteady. If you were suddenly dizzy, where could you find support to steady yourself? Walk through the space and ask yourself, is everything in here absolutely necessary? Increased space gives you the widest margin of error.

C6 | **Home Modification**

Bed Mobility: Getting In, Getting Out, and Moving with Control

One of the most important and often overlooked questions I ask is: Can you get in and out of bed safely?

It's not just about getting up and down from bed. It's whether you can lift your bottom-heavy legs to get into bed at the end of a long, tiring day, reposition your body from side-to-side, and get yourself to sit at the edge of the bed in the middle of the night safely. Can you move with control, or are you relying on momentum? I often see people, especially when they're tired or weak, launch themselves into or out of bed, overshoot, and risk falling.

For caregivers, the concern is just as serious. When someone can't move their bodies themselves easily, the caregiver often ends up lifting or pivoting in awkward positions, putting their own back at risk.

This is why bed mobility really matters. Two of my favorite solutions are using half-bed rails and Comfort Linen's friction-reducing sheets and pajamas to give people their independence back.

Medline Bed Assist rails are great for providing support when someone feels dizzy upon getting up or needs something to push or pull from while sitting, rolling, or standing.

A little tip here as I've had families call me understandably puzzled. "How is Dad supposed to get his legs over this bar?!" Those rails should be installed up near the pillow, not in the middle of the bed like the picture on the box might suggest ☺

When installed properly, with the safety strap secured around the box spring to prevent shifting or entrapment, the rail is incredibly effective at preventing someone from rolling off the bed and getting wedged between the bed and the nightstand, a really common cause of falls.

Comfort Linen is one of my favorite tools for improving bed mobility, especially for people living with Parkinson's. It helps them move more easily in bed despite stiffness. The sheets have a smooth satin

Age in Place or Find a New Space

panel in the middle that allows the legs to glide in and out of bed with less effort, which also reduces physical strain on caregivers. The edges are made from traditional fabric, which acts as a natural stopping point to prevent sliding too far or falling out of bed.

Another common question I get is: *What's the right bed height?*

In most cases, a height of 20 to 23 inches from the floor to the top of the mattress is the sweet spot. This usually allows the hips to sit slightly above the knees, making it easier to stand up without relying on momentum.

But this is highly individual, and the best height depends on the person's size, leg strength, and balance. What matters most is that the bed is firm and supportive, and that it doesn't collapse at the edges. A bed that sinks too much at the edge can make it harder to push off and increases the risk of sliding right off the bed when seated, especially after a hospitalization when a person's quadriceps may be too weak to support their body weight.

Sometimes, I recommend adding grip tape in a contrasting color on the floor next to the bed to help prevent the feet from slipping out from under someone when they're standing up. This is especially useful for people who are not used to shifting their body weight onto their legs to stand.

But it's not just about equipment. It's also about teaching the right movement strategies. One of my favorite biomechanics cues is to remind people: "Nose over toes." This helps them remember to shift their weight forward enough to unweight their bottom. I then encourage them to "Stick your bottom up in the air!" to allow the knees to straighten more easily, which is especially useful for those with weak quadriceps.

Safe bed transfers aren't just about preserving independence. They're about protecting caregivers, preventing injuries, and making everyday routines safer and more manageable.

When you can create a bedroom setup that supports safe, controlled movement, you reduce one of the most common sources of falls: getting up in the middle of the night to go to the bathroom. Thoughtful design here pays dividends.

Master Closet

Let's peek into the closet— when it's an organized space, it's not usually a fall risk. When it's crammed full of clothes, people need to bend, stretch, and balance on tiptoe to find what they are looking for, and it can increase their risk of falls.

Closets are full of micro-decisions that pile up quickly: reaching for hangers, bending for shoes, stretching to get something off the top shelf. These little moments don't seem like a big deal…until they are. I've had more than one client fall backwards in the closet when trying to get a suitcase down from the upper shelves or falling when trying to put on pants in a cramped walk-in closet.

What I'm Looking For

- **Shelf height:** Are everyday items accessible without a stool?
- **Rod placement:** Is clothing hung too high or too deep into corners?
- **Floor space:** Is there room to stand, turn, or sit while dressing?
- **Lighting:** Is the closet well-lit enough to clearly see clothing and shoes?
- **Shoe storage:** Are shoes loose on the floor (tripping hazard)?
- **Clutter:** Are there bins, bags, or boxes making movement difficult?

Age in Place or Find a New Space

Quick DIY Wins

- ☐ Lower hanging rods or use double-rod closet organizers to bring clothes within easy reach.
- ☐ Install motion-activated LED lighting strips or battery-operated puck lights (*Brilliant Evolution* or *GE*) to improve visibility.
- ☐ Add a dressing stool or small chair for seated dressing or a place to catch your breath.
- ☐ Use hanging organizers for shoes and daily items instead of storing them on the floor.
- ☐ Rotate seasonal clothes so current needs are front and center—store the rest in labeled, easy-to-access bins.
- ☐ Keep a grabber tool inside the closet to safely reach dropped or high-up items.

When to Call a Pro

- √ Install a custom closet system with adjustable shelving and rods at accessible heights (look for systems from *ClosetMaid* or *EasyClosets*).
- √ Install a manual or motorized pull-down rod (like *Granberg*) to maximize storage in a tall closet.
- √ Reconfigure a walk-in closet with sliding doors, wider pathways, or built-in bench seating.
- √ Add task lighting on a switch or motion sensor if natural light is limited or nonexistent.

Homeowner/Caregiver Self-Audit

- ☐ Can I reach everyday clothing without stretching or using a stool?
- ☐ Are my shoes stored off the floor and easy to access?
- ☐ Is there a place to sit while dressing or choosing clothes?
- ☐ Is the closet well-lit, even during the evening?
- ☐ Are the floor and path clear of bins, boxes, or laundry piles?

C6 | Home Modification

☐ Do I dread using the closet because it feels overwhelming or difficult?

#OTBrain Insight

Organize your closet in a way that makes sense to your brain. Your goal is to decrease the need to search or think too much. If you must get something from an upper shelf or on a stool, make sure that you are activating your core first before your arms go up, and be aware of the potential for dizziness when you tilt your head back (it will activate your vestibular system).

··

Future-Proofing: Building with Tomorrow in Mind

While we're in the closet, it's also a great time to talk about future-proofing your home.

One smart strategy I recommend during the building or renovation phase is to design closets that are stacked on top of each other, one on the main floor and one directly below. This is a subtle, cost-effective way to create the option of converting that space into a home elevator later if it's ever needed.

But here's the catch: it's not just about lining up the closets. You also need to make sure the space is properly blocked and reinforced to handle the weight of a good-quality elevator. Elevators, especially traditional metal ones, are much heavier than you might expect.

Don't get seduced by the sleek, futuristic one-person clear tube elevators. They're often cheaper upfront, but in my experience, they're also cheaper in quality. They typically only accommodate standing passengers and may not have enough room for someone in a wheelchair with an extended leg, or even space for a second person if assistance is needed. Despite the cost, it's usually best to stick with a traditional metal elevator that can safely accommodate a range of situations and mobility devices.

Future-proofing is about making smart, flexible decisions now that can adapt with you over time. You may not need it today, but creating these options early can be a game-changer later, giving you more time and more choices to safely stay in your home.

Master Bathroom

Now we're stepping into the master bathroom, one of the most important spaces in the house when it comes to safety and independence. It's also one of the most private, which means people can be reluctant to share too much information.

This is the room where slips and falls happen most often and where people are least likely to ask for help. I've had many patients who sat on the toilet in the morning and simply couldn't get back up. The majority of them didn't have their phones and they remained stuck there until family members returned home from work that afternoon. Sometimes it's due to leg weakness, sometimes a urinary tract infection that leaves them feeling drained, and other times it's general weakness after a recent hospitalization.

What I'm Looking For

> **Access:** What is the connection between the bedroom and the bathroom? Is it a pocket door that can be left open, or is there space for a magnetic doorstop?

C6 | Home Modification

- **Shower and tub access:** Does the homeowner prefer showers or baths? Is there a step-over? Is there a shower hose to use if someone is sitting? Is there a bathtub lift available?
- **Shower floor and walls:** Is it a non-slip flooring? Are there any visible loose tiles on the floor or on the wall that could indicate a moisture problem?
- **Shower bench:** Can someone sit if they were suddenly dizzy from exertion or an inverted head position? Does the homeowner have co-morbidities like heart disease or COPD where the heat and steam from the shower can trigger shortness of breath?
- **Shower Grab bars:** Is there a bar that can be used in standing for support when tilting the head back to rinse hair? Is there a bar to hold onto when stepping into the shower?
- **Water temperature controls:** Are they easy to adjust and safe from scalding? Is there a bar to hold onto when turning it on and off?
- **Exhaust fan:** Is there a working fan? Does it have a light? Does it track humidity?
- **Outside shower seating:** Is there a place to sit to dry off and get dressed?
- **Toilet room access:** How does the person access the toilet? Can a walker fit into that space or do they leave it at the door?
- **Toilet sit to stand:** Can they get up and down from the toilet without plopping? What is the height of the toilet? Are there grab bars to help them stand or to steady them when pulling up clothes?
- **Toilet hygiene:** Is there a raised toilet seat or toilet arms to manage hip precautions? Is a bidet available for hygiene for a back surgery patient who has no-twisting precautions?
- **Sinks:** Does the counter height work for the height of the people who live in that space?
- **Bathroom Flooring:** Is it non-slip, especially when wet? Is there a need for radiant heat flooring to help the space dry faster or to help people with neuropathy feel less pins-and-needles when

walking on cold floors? Would they benefit from an air-drying system like *Airmada*, an exhaust fan with heat, or a heated towel rack for additional sources of heat in the bathroom to dry the floor quicker?
- **Lighting:** Are switches within reach? Is it bright enough at night? Do they turn on automatically when you enter?
- **Storage:** Are toiletries and towels easily accessible, without needing to twist to see what's under the sink?

Quick DIY Wins

- ☐ **Use a non-slip shower mat** or adhesive treads on the shower floor. (I like industrial kitchen style mats with drainage holes that let water flow away from the feet—just be sure to remove them after each use.
- ☐ **Another option is to use *SlipDoctor* spray**, which you can easily find on Amazon. Think of it as the perfect blend of glue and sand—that's exactly what it feels like.
- ☐ **Add a shower chair** or teak bench that is higher than your knees + preferably with arms to push up from and reach back for. *Carex* offers an affordable plastic chair with adjustable legs that twist, providing excellent stability on uneven floors.
- ☐ **Use a handheld showerhead** with a pause button to keep water trickling at a warm temperature while you lather up.
- ☐ Install bathroom safety equipment like a **raised toilet seat** with arms to push up from (*Bemis* makes quality seats) or use a 3-in-1 commode frame (often easy to find at thrift stores but be sure to check that there is no rust that could lead to a peg giving way).
- ☐ **Install a bidet attachment** to manage hygiene needs after surgery and to prevent urinary tract infections with more thorough cleaning. Many bidets come with a female mode that adjusts the spray angle, which is especially helpful for achieving a better clean during menstruation. The installation is simple

C6 | Home Modification

using the two bolts on the seat. Note: This is for cold water wash only.

☐ **Install a motion-activated plug-in light** and a battery-operated light under the cabinet toe kick to safely guide nighttime trips to the bathroom.

When to Call a Pro

√ **Install layered lighting** for floor lighting, eye-level lighting, and overhead lighting. Ideally hardwired to be connected to a smart home system and to decrease the need to switch batteries.

√ **Install rocker or toggle switches** placed 36-42" above the floor

√ Install an electrical outlet if in an older home and want heated seat and bidet features (*BioBidet* or *Brondell*, or *Toto* are reliable options)

√ **Install a jet dry system** to reduce water on the floor. *Airmada* makes a quality one and also has a genius system to retrofit a shower into a steam room to offer a way to manage joint pain and muscle aches of aging.

√ **In the shower, install a vertical grab bar** to help you over the threshold, a horizontal one to steady yourself while in the shower, and a shampoo shelf or corner shelf grab bar to minimize the trip hazard of bottles off the floor and provide support when rinsing hair or adjusting the temperature controls.

√ **For clients who need more support**, depending on the size of the shower, I will do three long bars to make a circle of support or install a continuous reassurance rail throughout the entire shower.

√ **Install a dual-purpose toilet paper grab bar** in front of the toilet to promote forward weight shifting

√ **I have a signature L-shaped grab bar system** that combines a vertical bar for pulling up from the toilet with a horizontal bar for steadying yourself while managing clothing. When these bars

Age in Place or Find a New Space

are seamlessly connected, they create a cohesive look that feels more like an art piece on the wall than a safety device.
- √ **I like to put down a soft silicone grip tape** in a contrasting color in front of the toilet for extra safety with bare feet. (*Cat Tongue* comes in black, which is great for white floors).
- √ **For safety for men,** I will also sometimes install a horizontal bar on the back wall for stability when turning to flush who prefer to stand.
- √ **My favorite brands, according to price point, are listed below**: ** Note that not all bars are suitable for retrofitting.
- √ The ideal situation is for the space to be blocked for more options:
    - *Ponte Giulio* and *HealthCraft* have everything from **high-end to affordable**
    - *Great Grabz, Grabaccessories,* and *SeaChrome* have **mid-range bars**
    - *Moen and Delta* make mid-range to **affordable bars**
- √ **Install a zero-threshold shower** if stepping over is difficult. If time is a consideration, *Best Bath* has excellent quality, prefabricated ones, but a certified installer must install them to avoid mold and mildew behind the walls.
- √ **If funds are limited** and you don't need it to be completely barrier-free, a contractor can do what is called a **tub cut** which is an opening in the bathtub and place a water cover over it. You will end up with a 3" to 4" lip to step over rather than needing to lift the leg completely over the edge.
- √ **Flooring surface replacement:** If the surface is too slick, consider upgrading to non-slip, low-profile flooring. *Altro* is common in hospitals and now has beautiful consumer options.
- √ **Injury Prevention flooring:** If the floor is made of slick marble or travertine tile or if a fear of falling has developed, *Viconic* has an impact-absorbing underlayment that float over those hard surfaces.

C6 | Home Modification

Pro Tip: It can be installed beneath flexible flooring like carpet or vinyl, and when it's no longer needed, it can be easily removed without damaging the original surface. Ideal for preserving expensive marble-type flooring for future homeowners.

Homeowner/Caregiver Self-Audit

- Can I step into and out of the shower or tub safely, without losing balance?
- Is the floor slippery when wet?
- Do I have something secure to hold onto near the toilet and shower?
- Can I reach all my toiletries without bending or stretching?
- Is the lighting adequate, day and night?
- Do I avoid bathing or toileting alone out of fear of falling?

#OTBrain Insight

A bathroom upgrade isn't about aging. It's about safety and empowerment. If you hesitate to use your shower or struggle to stand from the toilet, your environment is asking to be changed to suit the person you are nw. Grab bars can be reused in a later renovation, so don't wait to put them in!

No-Construction Solutions: Adapting without Remodeling

While a tub-to-shower conversion is often ideal, it's not always possible, especially in rental units, multi-story homes with no full bath on the main level, or when planned renovations are delayed due to supply chain issues.

Age in Place or Find a New Space

In these situations, non-construction options offer valuable temporary solutions. When renovations are weeks or months away, these adaptations can immediately improve safety without the wait.

One of the most flexible solutions is a portable shower system that can be set up in any room with access to a sink faucet. There are several models available, but my go-to choice is *Shower Bay*. These units are sturdy, easy to assemble, and can be disassembled and stored when not in use—a great option for small apartments or families who may relocate in the future.

Other creative no-construction options include outdoor showers with portable ramps (great in warmer climates) and pump-action camping showers for urgent, temporary bathing needs. Sometimes, when all a person wants is to wash their hair, I've even used a 3-in-1 commode as a modified hairdressing station.

The reality is, aging in place is not one-size-fits-all. Not everyone owns their home, not every floor plan can be modified, and not every situation allows for a remodel. These portable, adaptable solutions empower people to stay safe and comfortable in their current spaces while waiting for the "perfect" renovation.

Luxury Accessibility: Why Beauty and Function Must Coexist

When I approach a space, my primary goals for home modification are to create safe environments that reduce the fear of falling, minimize home maintenance, and offer homeowners the opportunity to design spaces that truly reflect their tastes.

Throughout this book, I've emphasized the importance of client-centered goals, and as you might have noticed, for most people, the goal is almost always a blend of "I want it to work" and "I want it to be beautiful."

C6 | Home Modification

This desire for beauty isn't superficial—it's rooted in something much deeper. Our environments shape our emotional well-being, and there is powerful science that backs this up.

When people create beautiful spaces, they experience a physiological sense of calm. It's not just about aesthetics. It's about feeling safe, at ease, and proud of their home.

At Evolving Homes®, this is something we truly care about. Over the years, I've learned how important it is to find solutions that are both quick and beautiful. When someone falls, they don't have the luxury of waiting six months for a perfect remodel—they need something that works right now. But just as important, it should still feel like home.

This section is meant to serve as a road map for fellow professionals who may want to replicate or adapt these solutions. I want to share what I've learned in hopes that others can use it, improve it, and build upon it. There's so much need in this space—and the more we collaborate, the greater the impact we can have together. When we collaborate on ideas and work as a team across disciplines, we create safer, more beautiful spaces that truly resonate with the people we serve.

Here's the system I've found that balances both function and beauty in a way that clients really connect with.

The Evolving Homes® Luxury Accessibility Tub-to-Shower Conversion

"I know you'll be right next to me, but I'm just too afraid of falling again. I can't do it."

This need became clear through my work with clients who often resisted attempts to re-enter their showers. I designed this system to replace that fear with calm, confidence, and beauty. I wanted clients to feel empowered in the design process, giving them the freedom to express their tastes and the agency to create spaces that feel like home, not like a medical intervention.

Age in Place or Find a New Space

There is no universal solution, but this approach has provided comfort and reassurance to many of my clients. I hope sharing this perspective can provide you with a clear starting point for you as well.

Key Features of the Evolving Homes® System

1. **Ceiling-Mounted Shower Curtain & Rod System**
    - Inspired by hospital privacy curtains but with an elegant upgrade.
    - The ceiling mount prevents grabbing tension rods that can collapse.
    - Adds height, maximizes light, and slides smoothly.
    - Accommodates toilet-to-shower transfers and uneven walls.
    - Paired with heavy-duty clear liners to protect finishes.
2. **Premium Pre-Blocked Prefab Showers**
    - Made with gel-coated fiberglass (similar to Corvette exteriors) for durability.
    - Pre-blocked for grab bars.
    - Quick installation with minimal maintenance (no grout lines).
    - Customizable designer finishes.
    - Trench drains provide:
        - Consistent slope for safer transfers.
        - Better overflow control.
        - Sleek, modern look with customizable metal accents.
3. **Elegant, Sculptural Grab Bars**
    - Designed to look like high-end bathroom fixtures.
    - Includes options like toilet paper holder bars and corner shampoo-shelf bars.
    - Modular and interchangeable to allow future color or finish changes without drilling new holes.

C6 | Home Modification

4. **Movable Shower Seating**
   - Lightweight, repositionable seating for flexible support.
   - Stored out of the way when not needed.
5. **Mold & Moisture Prevention**
   - Pre-treated studs to prevent termite and moisture damage.
   - Humidity-sensing fans with integrated lighting.
   - Optional heated floors or air-drying systems to reduce maintenance and dry the space faster.
6. **Additional Features**
   - Heated bidet toilet seats for hygiene and comfort.
   - High-quality, non-skid flooring combined with injury-prevention underlayment.
   - Adjustable-height countertops for ergonomic access.

My goal is to challenge outdated assumptions that accessibility is bland by creating spaces that harmoniously blend both beauty and function. This is a powerful example of how safety and aesthetics can—and should—coexist in everyday living spaces, offering a thoughtful shift in how we approach accessible design for the future.

The Psychology of Calm

The field of neurasthenics shows us how beautiful spaces can have measurable calming effects on the nervous system and how design choices can shape not only our emotional state but also our physical well-being.

We all know that feeling—walking into a room that just feels right. Maybe it's the softness of the textures, the quality of the light, or the subtle sound of water. Whatever it is, your body knows it's safe even before your mind catches up.

So, when clients say they don't want their homes to look like hospitals, I understand. Cold, clinical spaces can increase anxiety. Warm, intentional design can create calm.

In her 2023 installation *Home as Self*, unveiled at Salone del Mobile in Milan, architect Suchi Reddy brought these ideas to life. Visitors walked through immersive environments while biometric sensors captured their physiological responses, monitoring heart rate, emotional markers, and perceptions of safety. The results were clear: environments that engage the senses holistically reduce stress, improve emotional regulation, and even boost cognitive performance.

Beautiful spaces aren't just about style. They impact how we heal, how we rest, and how safe we feel in our homes.

Biophilic Design: Nature as Therapy

Biophilic design embraces our natural connection to the outdoors. Incorporating indoor plants, natural materials, and views of greenery can improve both physical and mental health.

Simple additions, like the sound of running water or sunlight filtering through a window, activate the parasympathetic nervous system, reducing anxiety and promoting calm.

Even small details like wood grain, soft breezes, and exposure to natural textures can help ground us, can potentially reduce inflammation, and regulate cortisol levels. Many report a calming, centering effect that feels deeply restorative.

These concepts aren't just trendy—they're grounded in serious health outcomes. A landmark 1972 study by Roger Ulrich demonstrated that patients recovering from cholecystectomy (gallbladder removal) who had a window view of a tree recovered faster, needed less pain medication, and had fewer complications compared to those with a view of a brick wall.[xiii] It was one of the first studies to prove that our

C6 | Home Modification

environment, especially our *visual* environment, can influence physiological healing.

So, as you start to think more about the kind of space you want for your future, ask yourself: Does this space feel calm and comforting? Does it make me feel connected to nature? Does it feel like home? That's where design meets therapy.

OT-Built Platforms

Home for Life Design is a web-based application and service designed to help aging and disabled individuals live safely and independently in their homes for as long as possible. Designed by long time occupational therapist, Carolyn Sithong, it provides tools for professionals to assess and identify barriers to accessibility within a home and then track the effectiveness of modifications to improve safety and functionality. The core of the service is the Accessibility Rating, which measures a home's ability to support daily activities and tracks changes over time as modifications are made.

AskSAMIE is an AI-driven occupational therapy resource and marketplace, helping older adults, people with disabilities, and family caregivers find adaptive equipment and answers for developmental disabilities, aging in place and all the daily living needs. Created by Brandie Archie OTD, AskSAMIE also hosts OTConnected.com, a digital hub for OTPs to discover, save and share adaptive resources, grow their business and connect with a community.

IncluzIT HOME and **IncluzIT PRO** are two digital platforms developed by Canadian occupational therapist, Marnie Courage, CEO of Incluzia Inc. The goal of the platforms is to bridge the gap between healthcare and housing, focusing on accessibility and aging in place. IncluzIT PRO is a health and home assessment platform designed for occupational

Age in Place or Find a New Space

therapists, while IncluzIT HOME is a free, public facing tool for aging and home safety planning.

Final Thoughts: Your Spaces Through the Eyes of an OT

Modifying your home isn't just about checklists or grab bars. It's about creating spaces that keep you safe and independent. Room by room, we explored how to see your home through the eyes of a home modification occupational therapist. Every corner has the potential to support you or get in your way. When you make decisions with intention, you turn your home into a partner in your well-being. You reduce fall risks, lighten your daily load, and most importantly, stay in control.

You don't have to do everything at once. By starting little by little, year by year, you give yourself the gift of time, options, and peace of mind. Your home can be beautiful, safe, and supportive. And the future you deserves nothing less.

C6 | Home Modification

Key Takeaways

- **Entryway:** Eliminate tripping hazards and add lighting to make entrances safe and welcoming.
- **Living Room:** Arrange furniture to allow easy movement and reduce clutter that could cause falls.
- **Kitchen:** Prioritize accessibility by placing frequently used items within easy reach.
- **Dining Room:** Ensure stable seating and good lighting to support comfort and social connection.
- **Bedroom:** Choose a bed at an appropriate height and keep pathways clear for safe nighttime navigation.
- **Bathroom:** Install secure, well-placed grab bars and non-slip flooring to prevent falls.
- **Laundry Room:** Avoid cluttering the space above machines and always check for water or detergent that may have spilled on the floor.
- **Stairs/Hallways:** Add handrails on both sides and improve lighting for safety.
- **Garage/Storage Areas:** Declutter and use wall-mounted racks to minimize bending and lifting.
- **Outdoor Areas:** Use ramps, railings, and smooth paths to stay connected with nature safely.

Chapter Seven

Physical Fitness

Every home modification, whether it's a grab bar, a non-slip rug, or a ramp, serves one essential purpose: to prevent falls. In the previous chapter, we explored practical strategies to improve safe access throughout the home. But home modifications are just one piece of the puzzle.

Now, we turn our attention to another critical factor in fall prevention: staying physically active. You simply can't age in place if you're falling all the time. And sadly, it often takes just one fall to spark a rapid, life-altering shift—from independent living to institutional care. It's a stark reality, but it's one that can often be avoided.

The first thing most people think of when it comes to fall prevention is, *"We need to install grab bars."* And while grab bars are certainly helpful, it's a common misconception that they prevent falls. In reality, grab bars help you catch yourself when you're already off balance. What truly prevents falls from happening in the first place is building strength, improving stability, and moving with confidence.

C7 | Physical Fitness

Movement is more than just exercise. It's the key to keeping your world open and expansive. When you stop moving, your world starts to shrink. Sitting more, doing less, moving less—it all chips away at your strength, little by little, often without you noticing.

The importance of maintaining physical fitness isn't hard to understand. What's hard is overcoming human nature: the pull to sit when you feel tired, to avoid movement when it's uncomfortable, to slip back into familiar routines, and to underestimate how quickly the body can lose strength.

And that's the real challenge of aging safely at home: not just making the house safer but staying strong enough to live fully in it.

Falls Are an Epidemic

According to the Centers for Disease Control (CDC), falls are the leading cause of injury-related death among adults aged 65 and older. One in four adults over age 65 falls each year, with women accounting for three-quarters of all hip fractures, most of them happening in the bathroom or bedroom. Ninety-five percent of hip fractures are caused by falls.

A single fall *doubles* your risk of falling again, and after a fall, 50 percent of older adults permanently lose mobility to some extent. Falls in the older adult population are common, costly, and preventable.[xiv] And despite what many people think, falls are *not* a normal part of aging.

The Vicious Cycle of Falls

This is the heartbreaking cycle of falling. After a fall, or even just the fear of one, people don't trust themselves anymore and often rationalize that they should sit more to stay safe. It feels like the right solution: sit more, fall less. But the problem is, the more they sit, the weaker they become.

Strong muscles grow weaker, including the quadriceps needed to stand up and the pelvic floor muscles that support bladder control. Transfers from sitting to standing become harder and harder, which drives people to sit even more. The fear makes them start taking smaller, more timid steps instead of strong, confident ones, and soon, they find themselves spending five or six hours at a time sitting in front of the television, believing that this will keep them safe.

One common strategy to further minimize the need to get up is to restrict water intake. People think, "If I drink less, I'll need to go to the bathroom less." But this strategy backfires. When they drink less, the urine in the bladder becomes more concentrated and more acidic, which actually increases the feeling of urgency. They end up suddenly needing to rush to the bathroom, often waiting until the very last moment. As soon as they stand up, gravity pulls even harder on the bladder, and with weakened pelvic floor muscles, they are now in a race to get to the toilet before they have an accident.

This panicked rush, combined with the muscle weakness from all the sitting, leads to an even greater risk of falling. It's a perfect storm: weaker muscles, faster movements, and a body that is no longer prepared to handle the demands of quick action.

But the cycle doesn't end there. When people don't flush their system with enough water, the urine is left sitting in the bladder longer, creating a perfect environment for bacteria to grow. This increases the risk of urinary tract infections, which further intensify urgency and can also cause dizziness, confusion, and overall weakness that directly increase the risk of falling.

Dehydration also has another hidden danger. When there's less fluid in the body, there's less blood volume circulating. This can lead to orthostatic hypotension—a drop in blood pressure when standing up. People often experience this dizziness about ten steps away from where they started, finding themselves too far from a chair or stable surface. In those moments, they crumple to the floor before they can catch themselves.

It's a vicious cycle, one that begins with the fear of falling and gradually pulls people deeper into the very situation they are so

C7 | Physical Fitness

desperately trying to avoid. We'll talk more about ways to break out of this cycle at the end of this chapter.

∎ ∙ ∎

The Origin of Evolving Homes®

I founded Evolving Homes® in 2020 to offer solutions to these very challenges, problems I saw over and over again as a home health clinician. The skills and education I provided always centered on practical, sustainable strategies: how to assess and adapt a home for safety, how to create client-centered exercise programs that people would actually do, how to build positive aging habits to prevent hospitalizations, and how to reduce caregiver burden through smart use of technology.

I loved working in the home environment: side by side with patients and caregivers, helping them navigate the unknowns and the unfamiliar after a loved one's hospitalization. I thrived on the challenge of solving big problems with limited resources. That's the MacGyver in me—my #otbrain found real joy in coming up with creative, inexpensive, temporary solutions to get people through the rough patches.

That kind of hands-on, practical problem-solving truly filled my cup. It was a deeply rewarding and genuinely transformative chapter in my career. I often felt like I learned far more from my patients than they ever learned from me. The lessons they shared about life, perseverance, and love were priceless and they've stayed with me long after the rehab sessions ended.

When the System Changed

After more than a decade in home health, things started to shift when it was reported that Medicare was predicted to run out of money within a matter of years if it didn't take drastic action. Utilization of therapy was slashed. Rules were implemented to reduce waste. Checklists and red tape replaced holistic care. The services that I felt really mattered like caregiver training, family education, helping people navigate their homes were no longer reimbursed.

We weren't allowed to spend time on things like ordering affordable equipment or helping them set up contractor appointments. There wasn't a checkbox to talk through the emotional side of aging and the complicated family dynamics that came with that. It became a system focused on reimbursement for skilled services like doing arm exercises to improve endurance to bathe without shortness of breath. But it didn't address the bigger picture: How do you safely move in your home? How do you protect the caregiver? How do you prevent the next crisis?

At the same time, hospitals stopped having time for patient education. Case managers were forced to focus only on the bare minimum, *"Do you have a hospital bed? Can we get you out the door?"* There was no time for conversations about what families should expect, how much help someone might need, or how to make transfers safe.

I realized that families were desperate for guidance. They had big, pressing questions, and no one had the time or the system support to answer them. On a personal level, I felt the constant tug-of-war between my desire to do what was best for the patient and the rigid charting requirements the home health agency needed in order to get paid.

But I just couldn't bring myself to leave people stranded. Time and again, I would close my laptop, set aside the paperwork, and dive in to support them. But there were consequences to those choices because the day's paperwork still had to be completed, whether I stayed late in the patient's home or worked well into the night after I got home. Eventually, I found myself on a fast track to burnout, exhausted from trying to give the system what it demanded while giving patients the support they truly needed.

That's what led me to start Evolving Homes®. I wanted to offer people holistic solutions that combined both practical strategies and human-centered care. I wanted to support caregivers in the ways they needed to help prevent burnout. I wanted to encourage older adults to take

C7 | Physical Fitness

control of their health through movement and exercise. I wanted to inspire people to build positive lifestyle habits that would help them shape a different future for themselves, one that kept the important people and meaningful parts of life close for as long as possible.

Most of all, I wanted to empower homeowners to be confident and stay in charge of their own decisions. No one knows what they need better than they do, not even the experts. Professionals can offer advice, but no one should make them feel like their voice doesn't matter. It should always be a collaborative process. A professional's role is to educate and support the homeowner so they can make confident, informed decisions for themselves.

■■

The Cycle of Decline

One of the patterns I most wanted to solve was seeing the patients cycling back onto my schedule every few months. I remember greeting them with a mix of familiarity and concern: *"Hi, Mr. J. How have you been? I see you've had another fall. This time, you broke your arm? I'm so sorry to hear that. That must have been so scary."*

What's important to understand is that this decline didn't start with this fall or even the one before that. It started much earlier when the lack of regular exercise collided with sarcopenia, the gradual loss of muscle mass and strength that begins around age 35. People don't notice at first because life keeps them busy and the changes feel minor.

For women, menopause accelerates this decline. When estrogen levels drop, it not only speeds up muscle loss but also contributes to bone loss, significantly increasing the risk of fractures. Estrogen plays a key role in maintaining both muscle and bone density, and its absence leaves the body more vulnerable to weakness and injury.

As people age, they naturally tend to adopt a less active lifestyle with more sitting, fewer physically demanding tasks, and an increasing

Age in Place or Find a New Space

tendency to avoid activities that cause discomfort. The body quietly begins to weaken. Many people know they should make a change, but that time never seems to come.

Gradually, muscle loss accumulates. Joint pain starts to limit participation in physical activities. Posture begins to shift, subtly leaning forward or to one side, eventually compromising balance. Over the course of months or even years, strength slowly erodes. Life goes on, and most people don't realize they are inching closer to a tipping point.

Then one day, often during something as ordinary as a nightly trip to the bathroom, they fall. And that's where their journey intersects with mine.

The ambulance is called, the family is notified, and suddenly everyone is scrambling to book flights. The patient is hospitalized and, with each day spent in bed, their body grows weaker. It's estimated that a person can lose up to two pounds of muscle per day while hospitalized. The speed at which someone can go from being completely independent to lacking the strength to even roll from side to side in bed often takes my patients by surprise. The decline is swift, and it's devastating.

Once stable, they are discharged home with home health services, where they receive visits from occupational therapists, physical therapists, and nurses, usually two to three times a week for up to four weeks. They feel stronger and more confident in their steps. With skilled support, many patients regain much of what they lost, sometimes getting back to where they were before the fall.

This is great, but what happens when therapy discharges? During those four weeks, clinicians showed up at their door regularly for exercises, took their vitals, and talked to them about the importance of limiting sugar if they are diabetics and limiting salt if they have high blood pressure. They got stronger because there was a consistent input of healthy habits from external sources.

When home health is set to discharge, clinicians remind the patient and family, *"Don't forget, it's really important that you keep doing these exercises to stay strong."* The spouse often encourages them to

C7 | Physical Fitness

continue, but the patient typically insists, *"I'm fine now. I don't need to keep doing them."*

These patients just lost their weekly exercise visits and along with them, the serotonin boost that helped fuel their motivation to keep going. Without that regular rhythm, they often drift back into the same sedentary lifestyle routines that may have contributed to the original fall. Maybe it's sitting too much. Maybe it's spending hours in front of the TV. Maybe it's waking up late, missing medications, or skipping exercise classes because they just don't feel like it that day.

Little by little, movement tapers off, the exercises are forgotten, and the progress they worked so hard to achieve quietly starts to fade. The weakness starts and over time, the decline picks up speed. Strength erodes. Balance worsens. And then, another fall.

They're back in the hospital. And the cycle begins again: hospitalization, deconditioning, home health, short-term improvement, discharge, and another fall. Around and around it goes, each time a little harder to recover, each time a little harder to break the cycle.

Families feel stuck. Patients will flatly refuse to do the exercises with them, feeling like they are being pushed and controlled. Family caregivers are stretched thin, worn out from daily tasks like bathing, dressing, toileting, cooking, cleaning, and managing medications so adding making sure they exercise, especially when met with resistance, often feels like an impossible task.

Clinicians see the pattern coming but are limited by Medicare's rules, which prevent them from staying involved simply to maintain exercise routines. And the cycle isn't just about strength and exercise. It's also about information—what's shared, what's withheld, and what's misunderstood.

The Cycle of Misinformation

For a lot of the adult children who are on the receiving end of the news, the fall will often feel like it came out of nowhere. My experience is that

Age in Place or Find a New Space

people feel blindsided by the news, thinking that everything was fine right up until the moment it wasn't. This omission of critical information to the people who love you is part of the cycle that I hope to break.

Many older adults work hard to maintain the appearance of normalcy, not to deceive their loved ones, but to protect them from worry. I've lost count of how many adult children have told me, *"I had no idea anything was wrong. Every time I asked about the doctor's appointment, they just said, 'Everything's fine."* I've even had patients who fell in the bathroom and, when asked by an alert dispatcher if they needed help, claimed it was a false alarm, terrified that if their kids found out about the fall, it might lead to being placed in a nursing home.

Getting good information at the right time is critical, yet it's one of the most common missing pieces. And it's not just the family that doesn't get the full truth. When older adults arrive at the doctor's office—well-dressed, hair done, wearing their brightest smile—they'll often answer, "Everything's fine," and the conversation moves on.

But I know the truth. I see the behind-the-scenes effort it takes to make those appointments happen. I'm the clinician in the home during the mad scramble to get ready, helping the spouse gingerly maneuver the client into the shower and into real clothes after days spent in pajamas. I'm the one reminding them to bring the blood pressure readings we've tracked together and encouraging them to speak up about the dizzy spells they've quietly shared with me but haven't yet told their doctor.

I'm also the one pausing in those final moments, emphasizing again, the importance of breathing, pacing, and conserving energy. Because I know, from years of experience, that the effort of "keeping it together for the doctor" often comes at a steep cost. Fatigue is one of the most common triggers for falling later that same day.

So, what can be done? First, there has to be an element of bravery and willingness to look at yourself honestly and see what hard work needs to be done to change the course of this story. A fall is your body's signal that something is wrong and intervention is needed. The best thing to do after a fall is to take action right away and figure out the reason for the

C7 | Physical Fitness

fall. You have to get in front of it as soon as possible to prevent this from happening again.

The only way to get good outcomes is to start with good, honest information. One of the most important steps is having an open, honest conversation with your doctor. They need to review your medications, check your vision, and assess your balance system to see if there's anything medical that can be addressed.

I know this process can feel overwhelming for many of my patients, so I always recommend bringing someone with you to these appointments if possible. Having a second set of ears helps make sure you catch all the recommendations, and having another brain in the room can help ask questions you might not think of in the moment.

When families can't be there in person because of geography or work schedules, I recommend leveraging technology to stay involved. Ask if it's OK to use FaceTime or speakerphone during the doctor's visit so your support system can participate in real time.

I've never heard of any clinician saying no because even in my own experience, I find that having multiple points of view creates a much richer, more complete picture of what's really happening. Sometimes, it's an adult child who gently reminds, *"Dad, wasn't it when you were stepping out of the shower that you said you wished you had something to hold onto?"*

We've now explored the reasons behind falls and how aging in place is truly a team sport. Now that we're all on the same page, let's shift gears and focus on strategies to change the narrative. I'd like to share some conversations I've had with clients that have helped them recognize the value of making this a priority.

Protect the Life You Love

Let's talk about what strength really gives you. It's not about how many push-ups you can do or whether you can deadlift a certain weight. It's about being able to carry heavy grocery bags into your kitchen without breaking a sweat. It's about having the strength to lug a 30-pound bag of dog food because your four-legged best friend is counting on you. It's about walking across a sandy beach with your partner, holding hands, and not worrying about whether you'll lose your balance.

How would you feel if you couldn't do those things anymore? Would losing that independence change how you see yourself? Would you look back and wish you had done things differently? Don't live your life with regrets, especially when you have the ability to change that with what you decide to do today.

Physical Fitness is Brain Fitness

Most people don't realize that memory loss, confusion, and even dementia aren't just products of age. They're products of lifestyle. Yes, your genetics play a role, but your *daily choices* play an even bigger one. Cognitive decline is not inevitable. There is a significant number of dementia cases that could be delayed or even prevented by addressing key risk factors.

How can that be? Consider that movement increases blood flow, not just to your legs and lungs, but to your brain. That blood delivers oxygen and nutrients, fuel that keeps your neurons firing, your memory sharp, and your mood resilient. In fact, exercise triggers the release of chemicals like BDNF (Brain-Derived Neurotrophic Factor), which helps your brain grow new connections. Think of it as fertilizer for your brain!

And the good news is that you don't have to train for a marathon or live in the gym. Simple things like walking briskly around the block, balancing on one foot while brushing your teeth, using light hand weights while you watch TV, and taking the stairs when you can are simple activities that, when done consistently, build up over time. They protect your independence, your confidence, and your cognitive clarity.

C7 | Physical Fitness

Physical Fitness is like Money in the Bank

You know what exercise gives you besides strength, balance, and energy? Options. The stronger you are, the longer you can go without needing full-time help. The steadier your balance is, the less likely you are to take a fall that sends you to the hospital.

Yes, exercise can feel like a chore. But I encourage people to look at it differently: it's not just helping your body, it's helping you protect your wallet. If you invest $600 in a personal trainer, a gym membership, or some basic equipment now, that's a potential saving of $6,000 a month for care if you lose your independence.

So instead of seeing exercise as just another item on your to-do list, see it as one of the smartest, most empowering investments you can make. You won't be just adding years to your life, you're adding *quality* to those years. The more endurance you build now, the more freedom you'll have later to travel, volunteer, and make your own decisions. And you're giving yourself financial breathing room to live life on your own terms.

Physical Fitness Restores Symmetry and Balance

One of the most compelling reasons to choose physical fitness, especially stretching and strengthening, is to maintain left/right symmetry. This is something we don't think about until we lose it. Too often, people twist an ankle, spend two months in a walking boot while it heals, and in the meantime, their brain rewires how it sees the body. That awkward limp you developed while wearing the boot? Your brain starts to integrate it as your new normal. That's why, as soon as the boot comes off, one of the most important things you can do is start retraining your brain and body to return to balance, to remember your original normal.

The secret to my ability to spot a problem was observing people's bodies and looking for imbalances—differences in shoulder height, hip alignment, or the way one knee might turn in more than the other. What you don't want is to let your body accumulate these little imbalances over time. If you do, your posture can eventually become the sum total of all your old injuries, layered on top of each other. The more crooked things get, the harder it is to straighten them out.

One analogy that really clicks with my patients is thinking of your body like a car. What happens when you hit a big pothole? It knocks your alignment out of whack. And if you keep driving without fixing it? You wear your tires unevenly, and things start breaking down faster.

It's the same with our bodies. If you want to maintain your best level of function—if you want to move well, get more done, and stay active in the things that give your life meaning—you've got to put in the work to restore and maintain your balance. That means paying attention to tightness, stiffness, or subtle shifts that might be pulling you too far to one side. Addressing those imbalances now isn't just about comfort, it's about keeping yourself upright, steady, and moving forward.

Physical Fitness Breaks the Pain Cycle

One of the most overlooked superpowers of exercise is its ability to unlock the pain cycle. So many of my clients get trapped in this loop: pain leads to pain medications, pain medications lead to constipation, constipation leads to discomfort, and discomfort leads to moving less, which makes the body even weaker and the pain worse.

It's a vicious cycle, but here's the good news: we can flip it. When we start with gentle, consistent movement, something shifts. Exercise naturally releases endorphins, your body's built-in painkillers. It also stimulates digestion and gets the bowels moving, which helps reduce constipation and the heavy, bloated feeling that can make people want to stay in bed. As the body moves more, circulation improves, muscles get stronger, and everyday activities become easier, not more painful.

And there's another powerful bonus: you sleep better. Regular exercise helps the body tap into deeper, more restorative sleep—the kind that boosts energy, supports cell repair, and helps the body heal from the inside out. Better sleep means better pain management, sharper focus, and more energy to keep moving the next day.

Instead of spiraling down into more medications, more discomfort, and more fatigue, you begin to spiral upward into healing, strength, and vibrant energy.

Physical Fitness Can Inspire You to Be Your Best Self

Physical fitness isn't just about preventing falls. It can inspire you to become the best version of yourself.

Consider the story of Jimmy Choi. Diagnosed with young-onset Parkinson's disease at 27, Jimmy spent years in denial, leading a sedentary lifestyle that caused significant weight gain and reliance on a cane for mobility. His turning point came in 2010 when he fell down a flight of stairs while carrying his infant son. Though neither was injured, the incident was a wake-up call. Determined to change, Jimmy embraced exercise, starting with short walks and gradually building up to running marathons. He has since completed over 100 half-marathons, 16 full marathons, and even competed on "American Ninja Warrior" multiple times. Jimmy's story exemplifies that it's never too late to start; the moment you begin moving is the moment you start rewriting your future.

∎∎∎

My Story: Start Small. Start Today. Just Start

Here's what I always tell people: Just start. Don't compare yourself to who you were at 35. Don't compare yourself to anyone else on Instagram. Just focus on being the best version of *you* today. The goal isn't

Age in Place or Find a New Space

perfection, it's movement. It's progress. It's choosing one micro-action that supports your long-term vision.

Because like everything else in life—aging in place, making home modifications, building strength—it's not about going from zero to 100 overnight. It's about showing up. Being consistent. And giving yourself the grace to be a beginner again, even if you used to be an expert.

I know what that feels like.

In my 20s, I trained as a competitive swimmer, and in 1996, I missed qualifying for the Olympics by one-tenth of a second. That year, Canada was expected to take six athletes for the relay. After my event, I swam, took my drug test, got my rubdown, and waited. In the end, they only took the top four. I was fifth.

I'm not sharing this to impress you—I'm sharing it because I want you to know that I understand what it's like to be at your physical peak... and I *also* know what it feels like to be a million miles from that place.

I didn't swim again for 18 years after I retired. I told myself I was done being waterlogged unless it was in the shower. But in my 40s, I wanted to feel strong again. So, I got back in the pool. Same person. Different body. Want to guess how long I lasted? Five minutes. That's it. And I was completely wiped out.

It would've been easy to feel discouraged. After all, I used to swim 4 hours a day—240 minutes! Now I could barely do five. But I reminded myself: *this is just the starting point*. It's not where I'm staying. There was no point in beating myself up. I couldn't expect to jump from five minutes back to 240 overnight. That was my current reality, and I chose to meet myself there. So, I made a plan: tomorrow, I'd swim for six minutes. That's it. Just six. Because if there's one thing I've learned from being an athlete, it's that consistency is the only way to create lasting change.

So, wherever *you're* starting from, whether it's a brisk walk to the mailbox or a couple of arm raises from your recliner, start there. Start with what you've got. And keep showing up. Because if you do that? I promise you're already on your way.

C7 | Physical Fitness

Find What Moves You

When people ask me, *"What's the best exercise for me?"* my answer is always: It's the one you'll actually do. The one that feels right for *you*. The one that's going to stick.

Here's the thing: so many of us have tried doing what we *thought* we were supposed to do. We've joined gyms because other people did, signed up for classes we didn't like, or forced ourselves into routines that just didn't fit. No wonder it didn't last. Exercise is never going to stick if you're forcing yourself to do something you dread. The secret is starting with what matters to you.

What's the thing you want to protect in your life? Maybe it's traveling, hiking, playing with your grandkids, carrying your own groceries, or simply moving through your day with strength and confidence. When you connect exercise to something that truly matters, something that lights you up, it stops being about "checking the box" and starts being about building the life you want to keep living.

I would encourage everyone to watch a powerful YouTube video from the Canadian Heart & Stroke Foundation titled, "**Make Health Last: What will your last 10 years look like?**" I show this video to all my patients to inspire them to take control of their lives. The last line is, *"It's time to decide."* You can find more information at **Makehealthlast.ca**

This video is a great segway to talk more about intention and about having fun in life. What's the point of life if you don't have people to share meaningful experiences with? Ask yourself: *What do I need to be able to do to keep showing up for the things that bring me joy?* What physical and cognitive skills do you need to comfortably go out to your favorite restaurant, play poker with your friends, volunteer at Rotary, or travel the world? This is the real reason we move—to protect our ability to keep doing the things that matter most.

So, what do you actually enjoy? Do you like being outside? Do you love music? Do you prefer moving with others or flying solo? Your preferences aren't obstacles, they're the key. They'll help you find something that feels natural, fun, and sustainable, not just for the next 30 days, but for the next 30 years.

Start with something easy to build into your life. You don't need to overhaul your schedule. I do heel raises and squats while brushing my teeth and stretch while watching TV. Small, simple habits add up. When you find what moves you're not just building a fitness habit. You're building the life you want to keep living.

Easy Exercises to Do in Front of the TV

These are simple, low-impact movements that can make a big difference if practiced regularly. Aim for a few sets during each commercial break or every 15–20 minutes if you're streaming.

1. Sit-to-Stands (Chair Squats)

Why: Builds leg strength for standing up and improves balance.
How to Do It:
- Sit toward the front of your chair with feet flat on the floor, hip-width apart.
- Lean slightly forward and press through your heels to stand up.
- Sit back down SLOWLY and with control!!
- Start with 5–10 repetitions.

Tip: Use your hands on the armrests if you need to at first, but work toward using just your legs over time.

2. Marching in Place (Seated or Standing)

Why: Improves hip strength, balance, and endurance.
How to Do It:
- Sit tall or stand behind the chair for support.
- Lift one knee up as if marching, then lower it and lift the other knee.

C7 | Physical Fitness

- Try for 30–60 seconds at a time.

3. Heel Raises

Why: Strengthens calves for balance and walking stability.
How to Do It:
- Stand behind the chair, holding the backrest for support.
- Lift your heels off the ground so you're standing on your toes.
- Slowly lower back down.
- Start with 10–15 repetitions.

4. Seated Leg Extensions

Why: Strengthens the muscles that help you stand and climb stairs.
How to Do It:
- Sit tall in your chair.
- Straighten one leg out in front of you, hold for 2–3 seconds, then lower it back down.
- Alternate legs for 10–15 repetitions per side.

5. Side-to-Side Steps

Why: Builds hip and thigh strength and improves lateral stability (which helps prevent falls).
How to Do It:
- Stand with feet together, holding the back of the chair if needed.
- Step to the right, then bring your feet back together.
- Step to the left, then bring your feet back together.
- Repeat for about 30 seconds.

6. Ankle Pumps

Why: Helps with circulation and keeps ankles mobile.
How to Do It:
- Sit comfortably in your chair.
- Point your toes forward, then pull them back toward you.
- Keep alternating for 20–30 seconds.

7. Seated Arm Reaches (Core Activation)

Why: Engages core muscles and promotes good posture.
How to Do It:
- Sit tall in your chair with feet flat on the floor.
- Reach one arm up toward the ceiling while gently twisting your torso.
- Return to center and repeat on the other side.
- Do 10 repetitions per side.

Pro Tip: Make It a Habit
Try doing one or two exercises during each commercial break or between episodes. Little by little, these moments add up to stronger muscles and better balance.

Combining Exercise with Fun

Incorporating innovative approaches can make exercise more enjoyable, sustainable, and something you genuinely look forward to. When you blend movement with fun, social interaction, and even a touch of adventure, you're not just working out—you're creating experiences.

By aligning physical activity with your personal interests and meaningful connections, you're far more likely to stay committed and enjoy the long-term benefits. Here are some of my favorite ideas:

C7 | Physical Fitness

1. Gamify Your Workouts with LudoFit

LudoFit transforms exercise into an immersive gaming experience. Using your device's camera, it tracks your movements as you virtually ski in Italy, cycle the Tour de France, or raft in Chile. The app adjusts to your fitness level, offering both seated and standing options, making it accessible for various abilities. Its interactive nature keeps you engaged, making workouts feel less like a chore and more like an adventure!

2. Connect and Move with Team Vivo

Team Vivo offers live, small-group exercise classes via Zoom, focusing on strength, balance, and mobility. With a maximum of eight participants per class, trainers provide personalized attention, ensuring exercises are tailored to your needs. Beyond physical benefits, the camaraderie and accountability fostered in these sessions often become the highlight, encouraging consistent participation.

3. Explore the World with Virtual Biking

For those who love to travel, **Bike Labyrinth** offers a unique way to explore new places while exercising. You can cycle through over 800 virtual routes from your stationary bike, choosing your path at intersections to make each ride your own adventure. You can even record personal routes, allowing you to bike through familiar neighborhoods or cherished vacation spots. This interactive experience not only keeps you moving but also stimulates the mind, making it especially valuable for reminiscence therapy. Time flies when you're fully immersed in the journey.

4. Embrace Social Fitness Activities

Combining exercise with social interaction can significantly boost motivation. Consider activities like **Urban Poling** (Nordic walking), where groups meet to walk and chat, turning workouts into social events. Similarly, joining local walking clubs or group fitness classes can provide both physical benefits and a sense of community.

How to Ditch the Cycle of Vicious Falls

There's always something you can do to help yourself not to fall.

Move a Little More Every Day

First, don't wait until you feel strong to start moving. You get strong *by moving*. Set a timer to get up every hour, even if it's just to stand, stretch, or walk to the next room. Practice walking to and from the bathroom to make this feel like an easier task.

Stop Skipping Water

Please, don't restrict your water. I know the goal is to avoid those urgent bathroom trips, but drinking less actually makes the urgency worse. Your bladder does much better when it's consistently flushed with water. Start by adding a few extra sips each hour instead of chugging a full glass all at once.

Bladder Training Works

Your bladder can actually learn. When you stay on a schedule, like going to the bathroom every two to three hours instead of waiting until you're desperate, you can train your body to have less urgency.

C7 | Physical Fitness

Build Strength for the Bathroom Rush

We can't always predict when nature will call, so building strength and balance is your safety net. Exercises like sit-to-stands, mini-squats, and side-stepping help you move more confidently and quickly when you need to. Start with a timer to get up from a chair and walk to the bathroom every hour for exercise and then make it a habit to empty your bladder every two hours.

Keep Your Blood Pressure Steady

To help prevent that dizzy drop in blood pressure, keep your body well-hydrated and give yourself time when standing up. My rule is generally to count to 10 before you start moving to make sure your blood pressure adjusts. If you have been training yourself to get up every two hours to empty your bladder, you will hopefully have less urgency to move as soon as you stand up.

Final Thoughts

The strength you build today is the independence you protect for tomorrow. You don't have to love exercise. You just have to love what it gives you: your freedom, your life, your ability to be present with the people you love.

Let that be your motivation. So, what's one small step forward you'd feel OK taking today? That's your spark. That's your starting point. Once you find a little momentum, we can build from there. Every bit of progress matters. Because what stays in motion, stays in motion!

Age in Place or Find a New Space

Key Takeaways

- Your strength is your strategy—it's the key to living fully in the home you love.
- Muscle isn't about looks—it's about freedom, safety, and the ability to keep doing what matters.
- Movement is medicine for your brain, your mood, and your memory—no prescription required.
- Falls aren't inevitable; they're often preventable with strength, planning, and early action.
- Exercise is a long-term financial strategy—spend $600 now to save $6,000 a month later.
- The best exercise is the one you'll do—start small, stay consistent, and let momentum build.
- You don't have to love exercise, you just have to love what it gives you: dignity, energy, and choice.

Chapter Eight

Lifestyle Medicine

Throughout this book, we've talked about how your home can either support you or create silent barriers. But here's the truth: aging in place isn't just about where you live, it's about how you live in that house.

You can have the best home modifications in the world, but if you're not drinking enough water to prevent urinary tract infections, if you're not taking your medications on time, if you're not sleeping well enough to be sharp the next day—those changes can only take you so far.

A safe home without strong daily habits is like having a beautiful car with no gas in the tank. Lifestyle medicine is the cornerstone of comprehensive aging in place. If you're in and out of the hospital, relying heavily on paid caregivers, you're not living the independent life you've worked so hard to protect. Successful aging in place isn't passive. It requires active, daily choices that protect your health and preserve your freedom.

The good news? These choices don't have to be complicated. They just have to be consistent. And that's what this chapter is all about.

Why Lifestyle Medicine Matters

Most hospitalizations aren't caused by one big event. They build up slowly: missed medications, skipped meals, chronic dehydration, poor sleep, blood sugar swings, falls, unmanaged blood pressure, and repeated urinary tract infections (UTIs). Over time, these cracks grow until something finally breaks.

Here's What We Know

- Chronic dehydration can lead to UTIs, delirium, weakness, and falls.
- Missed medications, especially for high blood pressure or heart failure, can cause strokes, heart attacks, or hospitalization.
- Poor sleep weakens your immune system, muddles your thinking, and raises your risk of falls.
- Skipped movement leads to muscle loss and loss of independence.

When I worked in home health, I saw the same patterns over and over again. I met people who desperately wanted to stay in their homes but who were stuck in a cycle of emergency room visits and rehab stays. I met people suffering from swollen legs, struggling to breathe, or living with chronic confusion.

By the time they realized how much these daily choices mattered, their bodies were exhausted. They would have never chosen this outcome, but they didn't know how to change it soon enough. It's heartbreaking. But it's also preventable.

The Centers for Disease Control tells us that most chronic diseases, like heart disease, diabetes, and chronic lung disease, are preventable or at least delayable with lifestyle choices[xv] But too often, people spend the last 9–12 years of their life in poor health, bouncing between doctors, hospitals, and home health visits.[xvi] You can change that story.

C8 | Lifestyle Medicine

Obstacles and Mindset Shifts

So much can be done when we can approach things from a different perspective. I often hear things like:

- "I don't like drinking water."
- "I'm too tired to exercise today."
- "I know I should go to bed, but I just want to finish this episode."

In my practice, I ask people to see if this thinking feels different if we see it like this instead:

- You're not doing these things for today's version of you—you're doing them for your future self.
- You're doing them to stay independent and out of the hospital.
- You're doing them to keep your options open.
- You're doing them to have the energy and freedom to do what you love.

Some of the strategies I've found to make these habits easier include:

- Flavoring water with tea bags or fruit to make hydration more enjoyable.
- Use hydration monitoring tools like *Hydrostasis* wearable hydration trackers
- For people who need objective data to drive motivation, *TrueLoo by Toi Labs* smart toilet seats can measure progress.
- Habit-tracking apps like *Streaks or Habitica* can make it fun by gamifying your routine.

Your Habits Are Your Medicine

You don't need a perfect life overhaul. You need steady, daily habits that protect you over time. You need:

- **Hydration** to keep your organs functioning and prevent UTIs.
- **Medication routines** to manage blood pressure, cholesterol, and chronic illness.
- **Movement** to stay strong enough to avoid falls.
- **Quality food** to support your body and your mood. [xvii]
- **Sleep** to restore your brain and your energy.
- **Social connection** to keep your life meaningful and your spirit alive.

Taking control of your health makes a difference in your health. Here's what I encourage clients to build into their routines:

- **Get up at the same time every day.** It stabilizes your body's natural rhythms.
- **Take your medications on time**. Use alarms, apps, or visual checklists.
- **Drink enough water.** Flavor it, track it, or use hydration aids like Jelly Drops or Hydro Gummies.
- **Go to bed early**. Your body does its most important healing work while you sleep.
- **Move every day.** Walk during TV commercials. Stretch in bed before you get up. Use virtual fitness classes to stay accountable.
- **Eat more anti-inflammatory foods** that protect your gut, your heart, and your mood.
- **Stay socially connected**. Loneliness can be as harmful to your health as smoking 15 cigarettes a day.
- **Pursue joy.** Whether it's gardening, playing games, or traveling virtually, find something that makes you light up.

The Power of Routines

Routines protect your mental energy. It's why some school systems use uniforms, why presidents wear the same suit every day. It reduces decision fatigue so you can focus on what matters. When your habits are automatic, you save your brainpower for the big things. But when every day is filled with tiny, nagging decisions, "Did I take my meds? Am I drinking enough? When should I exercise?" you burn through your mental energy fast.

Occupational therapists use this strategy with people recovering from brain injuries all the time: simplify, systematize, and make it automatic. **I use this in my own life:**

- I keep separate packing lists for road trips and air travel so I don't have to remember from scratch.
- I use a grocery list with all my frequent items already written out—I just highlight what I need that week.
- I use store apps to find aisle locations so I can shop quickly.
- I automate what I can with subscription services that save time and decision-making.

Design your life to make the right thing easy to do. Other OT strategies I like to use for clients are:

- Daily checklists for meds, hydration, and exercise.
- Smart pill dispensers and reminder apps.
- Organizing your environment to support your routines.
- Balancing activity and rest to conserve energy throughout the day.

Building Micro-Habits

When life gets busy and motivation fails, micro-habits keep you moving forward. These are tiny changes that build momentum. The easiest way to build a habit? Stack it onto something you already do:

Age in Place or Find a New Space

- Drink water after brushing your teeth.
- Do a few stretches while the coffee is brewing.
- Take your meds right after your morning walk.

Here's one I've added recently: I keep stretching bands next to my bed and stretch before I even get up. It started as a micro-habit. Now it's automatic! What could you start with this week?

- Add a glass of water to your breakfast.
- Walk around the room during commercial breaks.
- Set an alarm to put your phone down at night.
- Snack on protein like nuts or yogurt instead of chips.

Start with one habit. Track it. Ask a buddy to help. Celebrate when you keep the streak alive!

Tech That Helps You Succeed

Don't forget, technology is your friend. Here are some easy examples:

Hydration Aids

- **Jelly Drops:** Sugar-free, colorful water treats that encourage hydration, especially for people with dementia. Available today and comes in 6 flavors like lemon, orange, grape.
- **Hydro Gummy:** 'Water you can Eat' Water-based gummies to make hydration easier and tastier. These are still in development but will have exotic flavors like Yuzu!
- **TrueLoo® by Toi Labs:** Smart toilet seat that tracks hydration and other health markers.
- **Hydrostasis GECA™ Watch:** Wearable hydration tracker that uses AI for personalized alerts.

C8 | Lifestyle Medicine

Social Engagement

- **Papa:** On-demand companion service connecting older adults with "Papa Pals" for social visits, transportation, and everyday support.
- **GetSetUp:** Virtual learning platform offering live, interactive classes that help older adults build skills and connect with peers.
- **Mon Ami:** Community platform that matches older adults with trained volunteers for regular check-ins, social visits, and practical assistance.

Exercise and Motivation

- **Team Vivo:** Small-group virtual fitness classes with social accountability.
- **Bold:** Online fitness platform proven to reduce falls by 46%.
- **RendeverFit®:** Virtual reality fitness experiences that make movement fun.
- **Mighty Health:** App designed for adults 50+ with joint-friendly workouts and nutrition coaching.
- **SilverSneakers GO:** Free fitness app for older adults, often covered by insurance.

Habit Tracking and Medication Apps

- **Streaks:** Beautiful habit-tracking app to build consistent streaks.
- **Habitica:** Turns your habits into a fun game.
- **Loop Habit Tracker:** Free, simple app to track habits offline.
- **MediSafe:** Medication app that can alert family if a dose is missed.
- **DoseHealth:** Portable, non-WiFi medication tracker that sends alerts to family.

Urinary Tract Infections: A Hidden Threat to Aging in Place

Urinary tract infections (UTIs) are a significant health concern for older adults, often leading to hospitalizations due to complications like weakness and falls. Understanding their prevalence and implementing preventive measures is crucial for maintaining independence and well-being.

The Prevalence and Impact of UTIs:

- **High Incidence in Older Adults**: UTIs are among the most common infections in older individuals. A systematic review found that the global prevalence of UTIs in older persons is approximately 23.6 percent, with higher rates in women and nursing home residents.[xviii]
- **Hospitalization Rates**: In the United States, UTIs are the second most common type of infection in older adults, leading to serious cases that require hospital treatment. In 2016, there were 551.3 hospital admissions for UTIs per 100,000 adults aged 65 and over.[xix]
- **Recurrent Infections**: Recurrent UTIs are defined as two infections within six months or three within one year. Approximately 25 percent of older women who experience a UTI will have a recurrent infection[xx] Prevention Strategies.

Implementing daily habits can significantly reduce the risk of UTIs:

- **Hydration**: Adequate fluid intake helps flush bacteria from the urinary tract. Older adults should aim to drink sufficient water throughout the day.

C8 | Lifestyle Medicine

- **Hygiene Practices**: Proper personal hygiene can prevent the introduction of bacteria into the urinary tract.
- **Regular Bathroom Use**: Encouraging regular urination can prevent bacterial buildup.
- **Cranberry Products**: Some studies suggest that cranberry supplements may reduce UTI recurrence, though evidence is mixed.
- **Probiotics**: Maintaining a healthy balance of bacteria may help prevent UTIs.

Family caregivers play a vital role in preventing UTIs:

- **Monitoring Symptoms**: Be vigilant for signs of UTIs, such as confusion, frequent urination, or discomfort.
- **Encouraging Healthy Habits**: Support routines that promote hydration and hygiene.
- **Seeking Medical Advice**: Consult healthcare providers promptly when symptoms arise to prevent complications.

By integrating these strategies into daily routines, older adults and their caregivers can reduce the risk of UTIs, thereby supporting the goal of aging in place safely and comfortably.

Food Is Medicine: Building Calm from the Inside Out

Your gut isn't just about digestion, it's often called your second brain. About 90 percent of your body's serotonin, the chemical that helps regulate mood, is actually produced in the gut, not the brain.

When your gut is healthy, you tend to feel calmer, sleep better, and think more clearly. But when it's inflamed, you're more likely to experience anxiety, brain fog, fatigue, and chronic illness.

Age in Place or Find a New Space

Eating anti-inflammatory foods can go a long way in supporting not just your gut, but also your joints, brain, and mood. Some of the best choices include berries, leafy greens, fatty fish, nuts, olive oil, fermented foods, whole grains, and green tea. On the other hand, excess sugar, highly processed foods, too much dairy, and artificial sweeteners can work against you.

It's not about being perfect, it's about making steady progress. Most of my clients tell me they start to feel noticeably better, less anxious, more energetic, more motivated to move, when they shift toward more gut-friendly foods.

How to Make It Work

- Keep a ready-made grocery list so you don't have to rethink it.
- Batch cook anti-inflammatory meals and freeze portions.
- Use hydration apps to build water into your routine.
- Track your meals and notice which foods make you feel better or worse.
- Try Gut-Health apps like *Cara Care* and *mySymptoms,* which can help you track how different foods affect your gut health.

Final Thoughts: You Are the Architect of Your Life

Everything in this book leads here: When you build solid routines, you free up your mind to focus on what brings you joy. You reduce decision fatigue. You give yourself stability. And you protect your freedom to live on your own terms.

Aging in place isn't just about the house. It's about the life you're building inside it. The routines you create, the habits you stick with, and the people you stay connected to—that's what keeps you thriving.

Start small. Start now. Your future self will thank you.

C8 | Lifestyle Medicine

Key Takeaways

- Aging in place isn't just about staying put—it's about staying strong, alert, and independent through intentional daily choices.
- Lifestyle medicine means treating habits like hydration, sleep, movement, and nutrition as powerful tools to prevent chronic illness and avoid hospitalizations.
- Health-span matters more than lifespan; living longer only matters if those years are healthy, active, and fulfilling.
- Many chronic hospital visits—from UTIs to congestive heart failure—can be avoided with consistent self-care and medication management.
- The most effective "miracle drugs" are often free: clean air, quality sleep, movement, water, and purposeful routines.
- You don't need to overhaul your life—just start with one small, sustainable change and build momentum.
- If your home supports your independence, but your habits don't, you're not truly aging in place, so take action today to protect your future.

Chapter Nine

Technology in the Home

Beyond just physical design, smart home technology is becoming an essential part of aging in place.

When you're in your 80s or 90s, you may find yourself living alone, and one of the big questions you'll want to think about early is this: *How will I get help quickly if something happens?*

The good news is that technology can address many of these safety concerns. Today, there are countless products and apps that monitor the home using sensors, cameras, and even predictive technology to track movement patterns. Some systems are designed to provide peace of mind to long-distance caregivers, while others are connected directly to emergency response services that can quickly call for help if needed. Many can even be customized to contact a family member first, rather than automatically dialing 911.

But safety isn't the only thing to think about. Technology can also be the bridge to keep you socially connected. Your brain needs connection and purpose just as much as your body needs movement. Today, support

C9 | Technology in the Home

groups, educational programs, and social clubs often offer virtual options, allowing you to participate from the comfort of your own home. There are even community-driven apps where people take turns teaching classes, sharing their skills, and building meaningful networks.

Technology is a cornerstone of aging well at home because it helps people stay engaged in what matters to them. Those who genuinely thrive at home are the ones who stay connected, keep learning, and continue pursuing the activities that bring them joy. That's the real difference between simply meeting your basic needs and truly living a meaningful, purposeful life at home.

Smart Home Technologies for Aging in Place

Simple assistants like Amazon's Alexa can be very helpful for aging in place. They let you control things around your home completely hands-free, whether it's turning on the lights, setting reminders, or playing your favorite music.

For someone with memory challenges, a voice assistant can be a simple, reliable tool to stay on track with daily routines, like taking medication or getting to appointments on time. It's an easy way to reduce stress and maintain independence, all with just your voice.

When we combine universal design with smart home technology, we create homes that are not only accessible but also adaptable. These spaces make life easier, more comfortable, and truly support your independence.

Connected products can offer new ways to manage old problems. Instead of finding out your printer is out of ink when you are trying to get ready for an important meeting, you will get an alert from the connected printer that low ink has been detected, and you should consider ordering more.

How about the pets that we feel guilty about leaving on their own while we go to work? Doggy treat devices can let you talk to your pet through the camera and "give" them a treat when you say goodbye.

Age in Place or Find a New Space

Amazon Alexa is a great way to get started, as it offers a low-risk entry point into smart home technology. It's affordable, widely accepted, and completely stigma-free, making it accessible to just about everyone.

Smart Lighting & Security

Smart lighting can make life at home both safer and easier. You can set lights to turn on automatically when you walk into a room or have soft nightlights come on to guide you safely after dark. These simple changes can make a big difference in reducing the risk of falls.

Controlling the lights and activating the security system are among the most frequently used functions in my house. I'm so used to brushing my teeth, getting into bed, and simply saying, "Alexa, turn off the bedroom lights and set the security system." that when I'm traveling and staying in a hotel, I'll get all tucked in and then sadly realize that I'm going to have to get up, lock the door, and turn off the lights myself. ☹

My Personal Assistant with Infinite Wisdom

One of my favorite ways to use Alexa is when I'm in the middle of cooking and my hands are messy. It's so much easier to rely on voice commands than to stop and pull out my phone. I can simply ask Alexa what temperature to set the oven for roasting massaged kale or quickly get cooking tips without missing a beat. I can even have her play music to set the mood and add to the atmosphere I'm trying to create.

On Fridays, when I have a random mix of leftovers in the fridge, I can say, "Alexa, help me find recipes that include broccoli, leftover pasta, pulled pork, and parsley," and she'll offer ideas in seconds. It's also incredibly convenient on busy mornings to have Alexa play the news while I'm making coffee and remind me what's on my schedule for the day. She's like a personal assistant, always there to keep me up to date and help things run smoothly.

C9 | Technology in the Home

But Alexa doesn't just help me; she's heavily used by my kids, too. They each have an Echo Flex in their room (it's one without a camera) and they use it to set homework reminders, alarms to remind them when it's time to leave for school and use it to answer factual questions like "Who is Guiness World record holder for the most hotdogs eaten?"

Some of the most popular Alexa Skills for both kids and adults include *Jeopardy!, Song Quiz, Escape the Room,* and storytelling games like *The Magic Door*. There are also educational Skills that make learning trivia, languages, or math feel fun and conversational. The best part is that new games and Skills are added all the time, offering endless ways to play, learn, and explore. This tech tool is so much more engaging than passively watching TV. Alexa invites you to join in the fun and can quickly become a lively, interactive part of your home. With so much variety and constant updates, it's almost impossible to get bored.

Personal Relaxation Coach

Now, Alexa isn't just for fun and games. I use it with my patients as it is also a powerful tool to help reduce anxiety and support mental well-being. With simple voice commands like "Help me relax," Alexa can guide you through calming breathing exercises or play soothing sounds to create a peaceful environment. You can ask for a bedtime story designed for adults, which offers gentle storytelling to help you unwind at the end of the day. For moments when your body needs care, you can say, "Show me some yoga poses I can do to stretch out my back," and Alexa will walk you through simple movements you can follow right at home. These features make Alexa a supportive, low-effort companion that helps you manage stress and stay connected to routines that promote both physical and emotional health.

Age in Place or Find a New Space

The Brains Behind Appliances

Smart faucets take convenience to the next level by allowing you to dispense a precise amount of water using just your voice. For example, you can say, "I need six ounces of hot water in this cup in the sink," and the faucet will deliver exactly that. Brands like Moen's *U by Moen Smart Faucet* and Delta's *VoiceIQ* make this possible, offering hands-free control over both volume and temperature. This is especially helpful for people with limited mobility or hand strength.

Many modern kitchen appliances such as smart ovens, microwaves, dishwashers, refrigerators, and even coffee makers can now be integrated with Amazon Alexa for voice control and remote operation. This kind of smart home automation can be especially helpful for older adults. For example, a family member could prepare a meal in advance, place it in the oven or microwave, and later start the appliance remotely or with a simple voice command. Imagine having a frozen lasagna ready to go, and instead of navigating the oven controls, you can just say, "Alexa, start the oven," or have your family start it for you from wherever they are. It's a practical way to make cooking safer, easier, and more accessible, allowing older adults to enjoy more independence without giving up support from loved ones.

Controlling Your Labrador Retriever

Labrador Robotics has some of my favorite consumer-grade assistive robots. They are basically a smart rolling cart, but are truly a game changer for moving items around the house, especially if you use a walker, wheelchair, or simply don't have the physical strength to carry things safely.

For example, imagine you've just come home from grocery shopping, and you're exhausted. You can use Alexa to summon the Labrador to the garage, load your shopping bags onto the cart, and then tell Alexa to send it to the kitchen. The robot will patiently wait there while you make your way from the car to the kitchen at your own pace.

C9 | Technology in the Home

It's also incredibly helpful for transporting bulky items, such as laundry baskets. Instead of making several tiring trips carrying small loads on your walker or rollator seat, you can place a full basket on the Labrador and send it directly to the laundry room, keeping your hands free to safely walk or roll.

One of the best features is that the platform can be raised or lowered to your ideal working height. I usually recommend working at waist level to protect your back, especially when transferring clothes from the dryer to a laundry basket.

This height adjustment also makes it possible to retrieve a sandwich from a mini fridge, slide it onto the robot's surface, and just as easily access a higher shelf to pick up a medication tray and deliver it to another room. It's incredibly useful for people recovering from injuries, like a sprained ankle, who need their pain medication delivered on schedule while keeping their foot elevated. The Labrador can literally retrieve for you, help you stay independent while you recover, and keep you safe by doing all the lifting for you.

Drop-In Feature on Echo Show

The Amazon Alexa Echo Show has a brilliant feature that became especially valuable during COVID-19. I began recommending that my patients living in locked-down retirement communities order these devices to place on the end table next to their recliners. It allowed their family members, who weren't permitted to visit in person, to "drop in" and appear instantly on the screen. It's like knocking on the door but even better because when you drop in, you can do it quietly. If you see your loved one is taking an afternoon nap, you can simply exit without disturbing them and try again later. It's a natural, easy way to check in, see how their day is going, and get a quick visual to make sure they're doing well.

Supporting Less Mobile or Bedbound Individuals

One of the most powerful benefits of smart home technology is the ability to support older adults, or anyone, with limited mobility, including those who are mostly bedbound. I once worked with a patient who had ALS, or Lou Gehrig's disease, which made movement extremely difficult. ALS can affect people at a relatively young age, and in his case, his wife worked during the day. There was no need to hire a caregiver during those hours because he could manage much of his home independently from his bed using his phone and Alexa-enabled smart home system. His setup allowed him to conserve his limited energy while still maintaining control over his environment. For example, when his in-home therapy team arrived, they would ring the doorbell. He could verify who it was using his app, unlock the smart lock with Alexa, activate his Open Sesame automatic door to let them in, and watch their progress on the Ring tower camera to know when they had fully entered. Once they were inside, he could shut and re-lock the door remotely, then use the two-way talk feature on the camera to direct the clinician to the room where he was waiting. This system allowed him to maintain independence, reduce physical strain, and confidently manage his home and care even while bedbound.

Automatic Environmental Regulation

People with spinal cord injuries or conditions like multiple sclerosis often have mobility challenges in addition to being temperature sensitive. They can benefit from automation that can make daily life easier, such as smart thermostats that can learn your preferred temperatures and adjust automatically, potentially in combination with automatic doors that can open to assist with temperature regulation.

Doors that open automatically when motion is detected will make their experience moving around in the house seamless and can help prevent falls, especially when paired with universal design features like wide doorways. Automated door locks and window shades add another layer of convenience and security with minimal effort.

Alexa Pre-Programmed Routines

Routines are voice-activated shortcuts that let you automate multiple tasks with a single phrase. For example, you can say, "Alexa, good morning," and your home can spring into action: the lights turn on, the window shades rise, the thermostat adjusts, and the coffee maker starts brewing. At night, you might say, "Alexa, good night," and your home can automatically lock the doors, lower the shades, dim the lights, and turn off the TV.

The beauty of routines is that you can pre-program them to fit your daily life, reducing the number of steps you need to remember and taking pressure off your brain to manage all the little details. It's not just about convenience. It's about building a home that quietly supports you, especially when you're tired, distracted, or simply trying to move through your day with less effort.

Hands-Free Calling

Alexa can be a helpful tool for hands-free calling, especially for people who have visual-perceptual difficulties, trouble navigating a phone, or mild cognitive impairment.

By simply saying, "Alexa, call [contact name]," the person can quickly connect with someone in their contact list without needing to look at a screen, unlock a phone, or dial a number. This can be especially valuable in emergencies when using a traditional phone feels confusing or overwhelming.

While Alexa can't directly call 911, it can quickly connect the person to trusted contacts who can get help on their behalf, offering a simple, voice-activated option that bypasses the challenges of handling a phone.

Age in Place or Find a New Space

Other Helpful Features You Can Start Using Right Away

- **Organization**: Set grocery lists, hydration reminders, sleep, and exercise routines. I always say the secrets to aging well—hydration, sleep, and exercise—are free. Most fall-related hospitalizations could be prevented with these three things, and smart home routines can help you stay on track.
- **Home Maintenance**: This is a huge one for aging in place. Sensors can detect running water, spills (especially important in cases of incontinence), or even flag potential slip hazards. Plus, they can track indoor air quality.
- **Personal Security**: Video doorbells, app-controlled locks, and voice commands like "Is my garage door closed?" or "Lock the front door" can provide peace of mind. You can even set automatic door openers for package delivery—open the garage, they drop it in, and you close it from bed.
- **Social Connection**: This is my favorite reason to use smart tech: helping families stay connected. Think about what we learned during COVID-19: baby showers, cooking classes, virtual lunch dates. These tools made that possible and continue to enrich lives today.
- **Telehealth and Exercise**: Another silver lining from COVID-19. No more transportation hassle or waiting rooms. Virtual visits are amazing. And with smart tech, you can also follow guided exercise programs, track sleep, and monitor water intake—all key for aging well.
- **Caregiver Support**: Virtual support groups can ease the burden of finding care and give caregivers much needed support.

Privacy Concerns with Smart Home Technology

For people who are concerned about privacy, **Josh.ai** offers an appealing alternative to mainstream voice assistants like Alexa.

One of the biggest concerns with devices like Alexa is that they are always listening and may capture data that can later be used for targeted advertising or shared across platforms. Josh.ai, on the other hand, is designed with privacy at its core. Unlike Alexa, Josh.ai doesn't store your voice data in a public cloud; everything is processed locally on your home network. This is a significant difference for those who are uncomfortable with the idea of Amazon or other tech giants having access to their everyday conversations.

Josh.ai also offers a more seamless experience because it uses microphones placed throughout your home. This means you don't have to remember specific device names or room labels. You can simply say, "Turn off the lights," and Josh knows exactly where you are.

Another major advantage of Josh.ai is its ability to understand a wider range of voices and speech patterns better than many other voice assistants. For people with accents, low voices from conditions like Parkinson's, or garbled speech after a stroke, this makes a huge difference. Josh.ai is built to handle natural, everyday speech, even when it's not perfect.

Unlike Alexa, which often asks you to repeat yourself if it doesn't understand, Josh allows for more variation and is less likely to get stuck or confused. This means fewer frustrating moments and a smoother experience where you can speak the way you normally do and expect the system to follow along. For many people, this flexibility makes voice control more accessible and much easier to use in daily life.

While Josh.ai comes with a higher price tag, many people see the investment as worthwhile for the added privacy, better voice recognition, and more intuitive control throughout the home. It's a system built for those who value security, simplicity, and a voice assistant that quietly respects their personal space.

Non-Wi-Fi Options

Smart home technology can feel overwhelming, especially when you find yourself troubleshooting frozen apps or dealing with a dropped Wi-Fi network. Honestly, how many times do we just say "no" to trying something new the second a password or setup screen pops up?

For many older adults (or anyone who just wants their home to work without extra hassle), non-Wi-Fi solutions can be a breath of fresh air. These tools don't rely on your home's internet, which means they're less likely to glitch, disconnect, or get hung up on software updates.

Dose Health is a smart medication dispenser that uses a cellular connection instead of Wi-Fi. It's small enough to toss in a purse and is especially helpful for people managing time-sensitive medications, like those with Parkinson's, where sticking to a strict schedule is crucial.

Lotus Ring is a wearable ring that can turn lights on and off with just one press—no Wi-Fi, no app, no learning curve. It's connected directly to a light switch base that just magnetically attaches and gives you instant control without fuss.

Hello Everyday has a plug-in sensor using radar, not cameras, microphones, or Wi-Fi, to track daily activity in the home gently. It works right out of the box, and sends alerts to give family or friends a discreet way to check in without being intrusive.

These kinds of tools prove that not everything needs to be connected to the cloud to be helpful. Sometimes the best solutions are the ones that just work quietly in the background. For many people, choosing non-Wi-Fi options can remove the frustration, reduce cognitive load, and make them willing to consider using technology as a care partner.

C9 | Technology in the Home

How to Get Started

If you're interested in exploring tech for aging in place, here's my recommendation: start small. Pick up one device and just play with it. Learn how it works and get comfortable using it. Take your time. Tech can be frustrating. That's why simplicity matters.

- **Start with one device.** Try a voice assistant for reminders and basic controls.
- **Automate one routine.** Example: "Alexa, I'm home" turns on lights, starts music, and adjusts the thermostat.
- **Layer slowly.** Add medication reminders, water intake alerts, or security checks.

How to Learn More About Alexa

There is a plethora of places you can go to learn more about Alexa.

YouTube and Product Websites

If you're just getting started with Alexa, YouTube can be a great place to learn at your own pace. The **Amazon Alexa YouTube channel** features numerous easy-to-follow videos that guide you through setup, key features, and simple tips to help you make the most of Alexa. I recommend starting with *Amazon Echo Dot with Alexa–Complete Beginners Guide* or *How to Set Up and Use Alexa*—both are great step-by-step videos for getting comfortable with the basics. If you're ready to go further, videos like *Discover Skills with Alexa* and *Get More Ideas on How to Use Alexa: Tips & Tricks* show you how to personalize your device and use it in your daily routine. These are free, easy-to-access resources you can return to anytime you want to build your skills or try something new.

Age in Place or Find a New Space

Best Buy Geek Squad

Best Buy's Geek Squad offers practical support for digital literacy and smart home setup, including help with buying, installing, and using devices like Amazon Alexa. Geek Squad agents can assist with selecting the right products, setting up devices, connecting them to Wi-Fi, and integrating them with other smart home systems.

They also offer in-home visits, in-store support, and remote troubleshooting for ongoing tech questions. For those who require ongoing assistance, Best Buy offers service plans that include device protection and 24/7 technical support. These resources can be especially helpful for older adults who are new to smart home technology and want step-by-step guidance.

Personalized Tech Support

If you learn best with one-on-one help, there are options to hire professionals to help you keep moving forward on your tech journey:

Candoo is a tech support service for older adults, offering remote assistance, training, and device setup to help them use smartphones, tablets, computers, and smart home devices. It reduces the need for adult children to provide constant tech help, supporting older users in staying connected and using digital tools with more ease and independence.

Carevocacy offers one-on-one virtual tech training for older adults, helping them build skills in using smartphones, video calls, apps, and social media. It emphasizes patience and accessibility. Carevocacy also provides Apo AI, a text-based chatbot that answers tech questions on topics like telehealth, smartphones, and password management.

HTA-certified Home Tech Integrators can help you design, install, and set up a smart home system that fits your needs. HTA certification matters because it ensures the installer meets professional standards for quality, reliability, and customer support. Certified integrators are trained to recommend the right technology, provide in-

C9 | Technology in the Home

home setup, and offer practical guidance so you can feel comfortable using your system.

Where to Learn More About Digital Literacy

Local Assistive Technology (AT) branch

If you're interested in exploring technology that can support your independence, your local **Assistive Technology** (AT) branch is a great place to start. These government-funded programs work like lending libraries, offering free 30-day loans of smart devices and assistive technology so you can try them at home before making any decisions.

AT branches are especially valuable in **Tech First** states, which prioritize using technology as the first solution to support aging and independent living. Together, they make it easier to find, test, and get comfortable with the right tools. You can find your local AT program here: **https://at3center.net/state-at-programs/**

AARP Foundation's Digital Skills Ready @50+

If you're looking to build confidence with technology, AARP offers a wide range of digital literacy resources specifically designed for adults over 50. The **Digital Skills Ready@50+™** program, supported by AARP Foundation and Google.org, provides free, hands-on training to help older adults develop practical tech skills. Whether you want to learn Google Workspace, Zoom, LinkedIn, or mobile payments, these classes are flexible and available both in-person and online.

Senior Planet from AARP

Older Adults Technology Services (OATS) is a nonprofit organization affiliated with AARP, dedicated to helping older adults build confidence

Age in Place or Find a New Space

with technology to improve their daily lives. OATS created **Senior Planet,** which offers free, live, and on-demand classes, instructional videos, and step-by-step guides on everyday tech topics like video chatting, online safety, telemedicine, and online banking.

These programs were designed to make technology more approachable and help older adults stay socially connected, improve financial security, and fully participate in today's digital world. Several physical locations across the country now offer in-person support.

AARP Community Challenge Microgrants

AARP supports local projects that improve digital access and expand digital literacy, especially for older adults. Past grants have funded public digital learning spaces, broadband improvements, free technology workshops, and digital skills programs.

These microgrants often go to libraries, senior centers, and local nonprofits, meaning opportunities may be happening right in your own community. It's a good idea to check with local organizations or visit **AARP's Community Challenge** page to see how you can get involved or benefit from upcoming projects.

Local Public Libraries

When exploring digital literacy resources, it's important to look locally. Many public libraries across the country offer free digital literacy programs that go beyond basic computer classes. These programs often include hands-on technology workshops, one-on-one tutoring, and access to online learning platforms, such as LinkedIn Learning.

Some libraries also offer innovative intergenerational initiatives where high school students bridge the digital divide and foster mutual learning by teaching older adults how to use smartphones, tablets, social media, and other digital tools. For example, the **Teen Tech Tutors** program at the Cornwall Public Library in New York and the **Tech Help**

C9 | Technology in the Home

from Teens program at Emma Clark Library provide direct, personalized tech support from teens to seniors. National organizations, such as **Teens Teach Technology** and **TechPals,** also partner with libraries to bring these programs to more communities.

Local libraries are a valuable, accessible starting point because they often offer in-person support and flexible learning options right in your neighborhood. They're part of a nationwide effort to close the digital divide and ensure everyone has the tools to participate fully in today's technology-driven world.

Helpful Resources to Protect Yourself from Scams

People can protect themselves from scams by staying informed, slowing down before responding to unexpected calls or messages, and verifying information directly with trusted sources. Scammers often create a false sense of urgency, but taking a moment to double-check can prevent costly mistakes. It's important to be cautious with sharing personal information, especially financial or medical details, and to be aware of common scams like fake government calls, lottery winnings, or tech support fraud.

AARP Fraud Watch Network is a valuable resource that offers free tools, scam alerts, and a helpline you can call to talk to fraud specialists who can walk you through suspicious situations. They also provide up-to-date scam tracking maps and educational webinars to help older adults and their families stay one step ahead of scammers. You can reach the AARP Fraud Watch Network Helpline at **877-908-3360**.

Life's Genie is a super simple app that helps block scam and spam calls by automatically answering any call that's not in your contact list. It's like having a built-in call screener. When someone outside your contacts calls, Life's Genie picks up for you and decides if the call is worth your time.

It's actually so realistic that once, when my son called me from a different phone, he asked me when I hired a secretary because he was genuinely confused. It's a great tool if most of your calls come from people you already know, but it can be a little tricky if you regularly get important calls from numbers outside your contact list, since all unknown calls will be automatically answered and sent to voicemail. For more information, you can check out lifesgenie.com or call their support at **415-539-0300**.

Let it go to voicemail. If you prefer not to use apps, just let unknown numbers go to voicemail and only return calls you can verify. This low-tech approach, paired with AARP's resources, can also offer strong protection.

Fall Detection Technology

Physical Indicators of Fall Risk

Falls among older adults can often be anticipated by observing certain physical indicators, providing opportunities for early intervention.

One such indicator is **grip strength**; studies have shown that weaker grip strength is associated with a higher risk of falls, particularly in individuals aged 60 to 75. This weakness may reflect overall muscular decline, affecting balance and stability.

Dehydration is another critical factor; research indicates that dehydrated individuals have a higher incidence of falls compared to those who are adequately hydrated. Signs like skin tenting, where the skin remains elevated after being pinched, can signal dehydration.

Changes in gait, such as a decrease in walking speed over a year, have been linked to an increased risk of falls, regardless of cognitive status. Monitoring these factors like grip strength, hydration status, and gait changes can aid in identifying individuals at higher risk of falling, allowing for timely preventive measures.

Decreased arm swing can be an early indicator of potential fall risk, especially in older adults. Research shows that reduced or asymmetrical arm movement during walking is one of the earliest detectable motor signs in individuals with Parkinson's disease, often appearing before other symptoms. Even outside of neurological conditions, diminished arm swing can lead to decreased trunk stability and poor gait coordination, both of which are essential for maintaining balance while walking.

Fall Detection Pendants: Help, I Can't Get Up

PERS buttons (Personal Emergency Response Systems) have been around for decades, and in my opinion, I don't see them being around for much more than a few more years. The technology is just way outpacing their usefulness, and based on my experience, I'm not sure how actually useful they were, given all the false alerts, the refusal to wear a pendant that advertised their weakness, or the lack of battery.

What amazes me most is how Murphy's Law always seems to show up in the worst possible moments. I had one patient who was the only one in my entire caseload who faithfully put her pendant on every single morning. But one day, she fell in just the wrong way and of course, the pendant was wedged tightly between her arm and her body, completely out of reach. She lay on the floor for several hours, unable to move or call for help because her voice was so weak. Thankfully, her daughter stopped by the senior living community at lunchtime and found her.

I had another incredibly active patient who went to the gym three days a week and had a very full social life. He saw no reason to ever put the pendant on that his kids got him, and so when he had the bad luck of slipping on water in the bathroom, breaking his hip, his pendant was in his bedroom drawer. Again, bad luck; his phone was in view but just far enough to be out of reach. He was extremely weak and dehydrated by the time he was found four days later.

Lastly, I had another patient who fell and had her phone with her, but didn't want to tell her daughter when she called that she had been on the bathroom floor for several hours and couldn't get up. She reasoned

Age in Place or Find a New Space

that if she told her daughter, she would end up being put into a nursing home, and since the cleaning crew would be there the day after tomorrow, she would wait, and they could pick her up instead. But of course, by then, she was far too weak to be picked up by anyone except the paramedics.

Why do I share these stories? It's to show that falls aren't as simple as they might seem. Sometimes it's not that someone physically can't get help—it's the fear of what happens next, the fear of admitting there's a problem. And there are plenty of times when a pendant isn't pushed when it's needed, or a voice-activated system wouldn't help if the person hit their head and was unconscious.

What about an Apple Watch? It stays strapped to the wrist, so you'd think it's a good solution. But I had a patient who made an active decision that he didn't want a whole-house monitoring system because he felt his Apple Watch was enough. Where do you think the watch was when he fell in the shower? That's right. Sitting on the vanity.

The idea that a fall detection system will automatically call 911 sounds great in theory, but in reality, most of these systems are calibrated for fast, hard falls, like the kind athletes take. Most older adults don't fall that way. They often "melt" to the ground as their legs give out, or they might simply slide out of bed and find themselves unable to get up. The watch isn't designed to catch those types of falls. I had a Parkinson's patient who was so frustrated because her Apple Watch would constantly go off by accident, but the one time it really mattered, when she tripped on a curb while walking her dog at night, it didn't trigger at all.

I believe the real future of fall prevention and home safety is in passive monitoring, where your home becomes your silent care partner. Smart sensors and AI can detect subtle changes in posture, step length, gait speed, and arm swing, all things that a human or wearable device might miss. These systems quietly track changes in vitals, walking speed, stride, and daily routines to detect early signs of fall risk, cognitive decline, or health changes, all without disrupting daily life.

C9 | Technology in the Home

But it goes beyond just monitoring. In the future, homes will not only detect hazards like water on the floor but will take action, activating radiant heat floors to dry it up, starting air-drying systems, or notifying a family member to help resolve the issue. The goal one day is for your home to just work quietly in the background, analyzing data and stepping in only when needed, not just to alert you but to actually solve the problem when possible. I can't wait.

Simple Solutions

As we've discussed, everything has its pros and cons. Apple watches are still my most commonly used solution simply because they allow you to have access to a phone if you fall when you are outside the house, like picking up the mail at the end of your driveway or at a communal box down the street. It has no stigma attached to it since they are so commonly used, so the adherence is high. (But please, keep it on in the shower. That's why it has a waterproof band.)

Cost is an important factor to consider. That's why I often turn to my MacGyver-style solutions, like using ten-dollar wireless doorbells to get a caregiver's attention or twenty-dollar driveway alarms to alert when someone is on the move. If you want something that more closely resembles the form factor of a pendant but without the long-term contract, I've seen ones on Amazon for about forty dollars.

Cameras Are Not the Bad Guy

Privacy is also an important consideration. I like having an Echo Show with a camera in the living room but using an Echo Flex (which is only the speaker) in the bathroom. I always recommend having one there because being unable to get up from the toilet is an extremely common problem in the morning. In most cases, the rush to the bathroom means they don't have their phones with them, so having technology there allows a person to call their family first to save the embarrassment of

Age in Place or Find a New Space

needing to have their neighbor or the local firefighters help them out of that situation.

Camera use has been seriously vilified in the last few years in favor of sensor technology that gathers data passively. But I think it's important to realize that there is a time and a place for everything. I can remember doing home visits even before COVID-19, when older adults would tell me how much peace of mind it gave them to have a camera in their living room. They felt so much safer knowing their family could see them instead of feeling all alone all the time in their house.

I also had patients with motion-activated cameras that would alert families when visiting clinicians were in the house, allowing them to participate in family training or have a chance to speak directly with the nurse about a medication or a need for a dietary change. This helped reduce the burden on the older adult instead of trying to remember the answers to "So, what did the nurse say when you asked her…?"

Personally, I loved having Ring Tower Cams in every room of my house and outside. They were especially helpful during COVID-19 when my kids were too young to have phones but were home, learning virtually. One time, they called me on the Alexa to say there was a stranger walking around in the backyard. The first thing I did was check my phone—I could immediately see that all the doors were locked, so I knew they were safe. To dummy-proof my life, I had also set my deadbolt to auto-lock after ten minutes, so I never had to worry about finding keys or remembering to lock the door. Then I started checking all the cameras to find the stranger. When I looked closely, I realized he was from the termite company, just doing their routine inspection. Without the cameras, I probably would have felt more anxious and been tempted to drop everything and drive home to check on them. The cameras became my eyes and ears on the ground, giving me peace of mind when I couldn't be there in person.

C9 | Technology in the Home

Camera-Based AI Fall Detection Solutions

Nobi is monitoring device that is designed to blend right into your home—it looks just like a regular ceiling light and works unnoticed in the background. It not only uses smart sensors to alert if someone falls, but it also has features that prevent falls in the first place. For example, it will automatically turn on the lights if it detects you getting out of bed at night, which can make a big difference in avoiding trips and stumbles. One of my favorite things is that Nobi cameras allow you to review an incident and assess exactly what happened in the moments leading up to a fall. That's important because understanding *why* it happened is one step closer to preventing it from happening again.

  KamiCare is another option I've seen that's simple to set up and doesn't need a big home renovation. It uses a camera that can distinguish between a real fall and regular movement, which helps reduce false alarms. It's especially helpful for people who want something straightforward. They can get alerts in real-time on their phones and even talk to their loved ones through the camera if needed. What's helpful is that if a fall happens and no one responds, the system can automatically contact emergency services. It's a practical choice if you're looking for something that works right out of the box and fits easily into everyday life.

Sensor-Based Technologies

There are many sensor-based fall detection options now available in the consumer market, and as a caregiver, it can be overwhelming to sort through them all.

  One important thing to keep in mind is that most sensor-based fall detection systems are not directly connected to 911. Instead, they typically send alerts to a caregiver's phone or to a monitoring service.

  Some companies are starting to partner with rapid response providers, but these responses usually go through a triage call center

Age in Place or Find a New Space

first—it's not an automatic emergency dispatch like pressing a traditional medical alert button.

These call centers assess the situation: sometimes, the older adult simply wants someone to notify their daughter to check in, and it's not a medical emergency. Other times, the call center might recognize signs of a serious issue, like a possible stroke, and escalate the situation to emergency services.

This step-by-step process is an important distinction and can also explain why some systems are significantly more expensive. Those with professional monitoring and emergency escalation typically involve higher service costs.

I've put together a simple list to help you get started on some of your own research. Each system offers its own approach, and I always recommend visiting each company's website to watch their introduction videos and see which one is the best fit for the problem you are trying to solve. Most will have a number to call so you can discuss with someone directly to help you decide if they are right for you.

The exciting thing for me about sensor technology is how the data can be grouped together to help you see patterns and predict behavior; it's not just about detecting falls.

Sensors can track patterns like whether the fridge is being accessed but food isn't being eaten, which might suggest confusion, or whether medication drawers are being opened on schedule, indicating meds are being taken. Some systems can even notice changes in movement, sleep, or daily routines that hint at bigger health concerns. Sensors allow us to collect meaningful information that combined with context can help provide insights to guide future care.

1. Chirp

       Overview: Chirp is a wall-mounted, camera-free device utilizing radar and thermal sensors to monitor movement and detect falls without compromising privacy.

C9 | Technology in the Home

Unique Value Proposition: Uses a combination of radar, thermal, and acoustic sensors to detect falls and track activities of daily living (ADLs).

2. MiiCare

Overview: MiiCare's MiiCube uses AI to analyze ambient footstep sounds, assessing gait and predicting fall risks before they occur.

Unique Value Proposition: Predicts falls by analyzing footstep sounds, enabling early intervention.

3. Envoy at Home

Overview: Envoy employs passive sensors to monitor daily routines, detecting deviations that may indicate health issues.

Unique Value Proposition: Focuses on behavioral changes over time to predict potential health concerns.

4. SimplyHome

Overview: SimplyHome integrates various sensors to monitor activities like cooking and medication adherence, alerting caregivers to anomalies.

Unique Value Proposition: Customizable sensor systems tailored to individual needs, promoting independence

5. Caregiver Smart Solutions

Overview: Offers a network of sensors, providing caregivers with immediate alerts and data on daily activities.

Unique Value Proposition: Focuses on lifestyle trends—like how often the fridge or medicine cabinet is opened—rather than just emergency response.

6. Electronic Caregiver

Overview: Combines wearable devices with ambient sensors to monitor health metrics and detect falls, offering a comprehensive approach to senior care.

Unique Value Proposition: Clinical health hub for home safety and vitals tracking, such as blood pressure and glucose levels.

Age in Place or Find a New Space

7. EyeWatch Live
> **Overview**: Utilizes motion detection cameras monitored by live virtual nurses, detecting risky movements before they occur.
> **Unique Value Proposition**: Provides the "Human Intelligence" (HI) of a live nurse who can verbally intervene and guide a senior *before* a risky movement turns into a fall.

8. Livindi
> **Overview**: Employs sensors to monitor activity and environmental factors.
> **Unique Value Proposition**: Bridges safety and social wellness by integrating a simplified, always-on video communication screen with background monitoring.

9. Aeyesafe
> **Overview**: Utilizes AI-powered cameras to detect falls and monitor movement patterns.
> **Unique Value Proposition**: Features an AI dual-mode that recognizes the specific "thermal signature" of a fall while simultaneously listening for the distinct sound of glass breaking or shouting.

10. Rest Assured
> **Overview**: Offers remote monitoring with sensors and two-way communication, allowing caregivers to check in and respond to emergencies, including falls.
> **Unique Value Proposition**: High-touch "concierge" service where professional human staff perform scheduled, interactive check-ins to provide companionship and oversight.

11. SMPL Technologies
> **Overview**: Provides simple sensor-based alert systems, such as motion detectors and door sensors, to notify caregivers of unusual activities.
> **Unique Value Proposition**: Offers a "zero-subscription" local alert system designed for caregivers who are physically nearby and need a simple, offline notification.

C9 | Technology in the Home

Tech Solutions to Solve Transportation Challenges

Transportation is often one of the biggest hurdles when it comes to aging in place. Losing the ability to drive or navigate public spaces can slowly chip away at a person's independence, leading to social isolation, missed medical appointments, and fewer chances to enjoy the meaningful parts of life.

The ability to stay connected to the community, explore new interests, and continue showing up for the things that matter is what gives life its richness. These tools and services aren't just about getting from point A to point B; they help preserve independence, spontaneity, and joy.

GoGoGrandparent enables older adults to access services like Uber, Lyft, DoorDash, and Instacart without needing a smartphone. By calling a dedicated phone number, users can request rides, meals, groceries, and even home services. This service is available across the U.S., Canada, and Australia.

SilverRide offers assisted ride services tailored for seniors, providing door-to-door transportation with trained drivers.

Onward Rides provides companion rides for seniors, ensuring door-to-door assistance. Their services are designed for healthcare transportation, partnering with senior living communities and healthcare providers.

Topp Flight offers medically trained travel companions for seniors requiring assistance during air travel.

Local Transportation Authorities offer flexible transportation services specifically designed for older adults and people with disabilities, often referred to as paratransit, demand-response transportation, or senior ride programs. These are usually operated by local transit authorities and provide affordable, door-to-door rides that can be scheduled in advance. The names of these services vary by region, but they typically offer rides to essential destinations like grocery stores, medical appointments, and community centers. Visit your local transit authority's website.

Eldercare Locator can help you find what's available in your area and can help connect you to senior transportation resources near you.

These services are a great solution for older adults who don't drive at night or have stopped driving altogether but still want to stay active and engaged in their communities.

Travel & Leisure Options

Many options are available for seniors when it comes to vacation and leisure activities.

Senior Travel Groups

Organizations like **EF Go Ahead Tours** and **Adventures Abroad** offer curated travel experiences for seniors, ranging from cultural tours to active adventures. **Senior Adventures** offers affordable group trips tailored to the lifestyles of senior citizens.

Vacation Rentals
- **Airbnb** offers an accessibility filter, enabling users to find listings with features such as step-free access and accessible bathrooms. Hosts are required to submit photos and descriptions of these features, which are reviewed for accuracy and completeness.
- **Elite Cruise Lines** partners with luxury lines like Holland America to provide specialized "dementia-friendly" voyages that include 24/7 RN support, dedicated caregiver respite sessions, and customized cognitive activities designed to make world travel accessible and safe for families living with memory loss.
- **Cruise lines** offer themed cruises catering to seniors, such as art and music cruises. These cruises provide enriching activities and accessible amenities.

C9 | Technology in the Home

Travel Newsletters
- **Travel + Leisure Magazine** lists various cruise options tailored for senior travelers.
- **Wheelchair Getaways** lists wheelchair-accessible Airbnb rentals across the U.S.
- **Wheelchair Travel by John Morris** offers extensive resources for accessible travel worldwide.
- **Julie Sawchuk's Newsletter** provides insights on accessibility and inclusive design.
- **Curb Free with Cory Lee** shares experiences and tips for wheelchair-accessible travel.

Home Support Services that Lighten the Load

Aging in place is about more than just staying in your home. It's about creating a lifestyle that supports your independence, safety, and well-being.

Everyday tasks, such as cooking, home maintenance, and managing medications, can become challenging over time. Luckily, a variety of services and technologies are available to help lighten the load, reduce physical strain, and free up time for the things.

Grocery and Meal Delivery Services

Access to nutritious food is essential for health and well-being.

Services like **Walmart Grocery Delivery**, **Amazon Fresh**, **Uber Eats Grocery**, **Thrive Market**, **Misfits Market**, **Boxed**, **Shipt** deliver groceries directly to your home, eliminating the need for shopping trips. **DoorDash and Instacart**, accessible via **GoGo Grandparent**, allow seniors to order meals and groceries without a smartphone.

For meal preparation, **HelloFresh** offers meal kits with pre-measured ingredients, while companies like **Chefs for Seniors** provide in-home personal chef services that cater to your dietary needs and preferences.

Catering and Prepared Meal Services

For those who prefer ready-to-eat meals:

- **Mom's Meals**: Delivers refrigerated, ready-to-eat meals nationwide, catering to various dietary needs.
- **MagicKitchen** offers frozen meals suitable for seniors, with options tailored to meet specific dietary requirements.
- **Silver Cuisine by BistroMD** provides chef-prepared, frozen meals designed for older adults. It delivers nutritious, pre-cooked meals to your home.

These services are especially beneficial for individuals recovering from illness or surgery, ensuring they receive balanced meals without the need for cooking.

Assistance with Home Maintenance

Maintaining a home can be physically demanding. **Ace Handyman Services** provides professional home repair and maintenance services nationwide, handling everything from minor repairs to larger projects. **Task Rabbit** connects users with local freelancers for home tasks and errands.

Additionally, some communities have programs that connect college students with seniors to assist with basic home maintenance tasks, offering a cost-effective and mutually beneficial solution.

Medication Delivery: Simplify Your Routine

Managing multiple medications can be complex. Services like **PillPack** by Amazon Pharmacy and **MedBox** offer pre-sorted medications packaged by dose and deliver them directly to your door. This ensures timely adherence to medication schedules and reduces the risk of missed or incorrect doses.

Space-Saving Furniture: Automated Murphy Beds

For those looking to maximize space without compromising comfort, automated Murphy beds are an excellent solution to having an extra space for a temporary caregiver. Companies like **Zoom-Room** and **Hide N Go Sleep** offer motorized Murphy beds that can be lowered and raised with the push of a button, reducing physical strain and making them ideal for individuals with mobility challenges.

Medical Care Wellness Spaces

One of the biggest trends to emerge since the COVID-19 pandemic is the idea of transforming a spare room into a dedicated wellness space—a place where you can move, breathe, and stay connected to your healthcare team without ever leaving home.

It's no longer just about yoga mats and meditation cushions; it's about creating smart, connected spaces that support both physical and mental health. Consumer Electronics Show (CES) 2025 really brought this vision to life with a wave of innovations designed for home use.

There are now tools like **StethoMe**, a smart stethoscope that lets you listen to your own lungs and send the recordings directly to your doctor—no clinic visit required. **Eyebot** introduced a 90-second, AI-powered eye exam you can do yourself, no appointment necessary. Smart

Age in Place or Find a New Space

hearing diagnostics are showing up in everyday items too, like assistive hearing glasses, making hearing care more discreet and accessible.

Home wellness spaces are also becoming a hub for personalized health tracking. **InBody's Dial H30 and H40** offer easy, at-home ways to monitor body composition, and their **InGrip Handheld Dynamometer** helps you track grip strength, which is a key indicator of overall health. These devices use advanced bioelectrical impedance analysis to give precise, useful feedback over time.

Withings introduced the **Omnia Smart Mirror**, which takes this even further. It's an AI-powered mirror that can perform full-body scans to measure muscle-to-fat ratio, visceral fat, and even ECG readings. It pulls in data from other Withings devices, creating a full, real-time health picture you can review during virtual doctor visits.

One of the most interesting tools I've come across is **Lumia**. It's the first wearable that can actually track blood flow to your head in real time, which can decrease the falls that happen in the home from orthostatic hypotension. You just attach it to your ear, virtually unnoticed, and it helps you spot what's triggering symptoms like dizziness, brain fog, or fatigue.

It's a game-changer for people living with conditions like POTS, Long COVID, or chronic fatigue. What I love is that it's been tested at places like Johns Hopkins and Harvard, so you're getting hospital-grade data in something simple and practical you can actually use every day.

A fascinating approach to sodium management is the **Electric Salt Spoon** by **Kirin Holdings**, which gently stimulates your tongue to make food taste salty without adding real salt—an interesting way to address anyone looking to cut back on sodium but still enjoy their meals.

These wellness spaces are quickly becoming more than just home gyms. They're evolving into personalized health hubs where movement, mindfulness, smart monitoring, and real-time care come together in one place. It's an exciting shift toward making proactive healthcare part of everyday life.

C9 | Technology in the Home

Diagnosis via Voice

One of the most fascinating technologies in health to me is voice diagnostics. Companies like Voicinosis are leading the way by using subtle changes in a person's speech to detect early signs of cognitive decline, including dementia and Alzheimer's disease.

I love this idea because it's non-invasive and can be woven into everyday life, sometimes even during a regular conversation. **Voicinosis** won the Audience Choice award at CES 2025 with tools like *Brain Guard Doctor* for clinics and *Voice Check* for individuals to track their cognitive health from home.

Other companies, like **Canary Speech**, are taking a similar approach but focusing on detecting anxiety, depression, and cognitive changes through voice during virtual visits or even phone calls. Imagine how powerful it would be to catch something early—just from the sound of your voice—without needing complicated tests.

TELL is a startup voice diagnostic platform focused on the early detection of neurodegenerative diseases like Alzheimer's, with a special emphasis on Spanish-speaking and underserved populations.

Unlike Voicinosis, which primarily supports cognitive screening and auditory rehabilitation through clinical tools and self-monitoring apps, TELL is designed to work directly through accessible platforms like WhatsApp and Zoom, making it highly scalable for remote and low-resource settings.

Compared to Canary Speech, which specializes in detecting mental health conditions like anxiety and depression, TELL zeroes in on cognitive tracking over time, using culturally and linguistically tailored assessments.

Voice-based health screening is a fascinating step forward—non-invasive, easily accessible, and incredibly promising. It's only going to get smarter, more accurate, and more widely used in the years to come.

High-Tech Toileting

High-tech toileting is transforming the bathroom into a hub for proactive health monitoring and enhanced personal care. These innovations don't require people to do anything and seamlessly integrate into daily routines.

Best of all, they decrease the work on a caregiver...my favorite.

The **Empower™ Clean Care™** toilet seat by Bemis exemplifies this evolution. Designed for individuals with limited mobility, it provides automated cleansing with pH-balanced sprays and warm air drying, promoting hygiene and independence. It has oversized color-coded buttons with the ability to customize and preset the cycle of wash, rinse dry, spray barrier cream. Its features are particularly beneficial in assisted living and memory care settings.

For health diagnostics, **Toi Labs' TrueLoo®** smart toilet seat employs optical sensors to analyze waste, delivering real-time health data that can be integrated into electronic medical records. This aids in the early detection of conditions like dehydration and urinary tract infections.

Similarly, **Starling Medical's UrinDx** device attaches to the toilet to monitor urinary biomarkers, facilitating early intervention for chronic conditions. **Olive Diagnostics' KG device** uses AI and optical sensors for passive urine analysis, detecting biomarkers for various diseases without user intervention.

These advancements signify a shift towards integrating health monitoring into daily life, offering non-invasive, continuous data collection that empowers individuals and healthcare providers to manage health proactively.

Challenges and Solutions for Rural Populations Globally

Rural areas around the world, especially in countries with vast geographic spreads or highly urban-centered populations like Canada, the United States, Australia, Japan, Brazil, India, and China, face serious challenges in providing equitable access to medical and rehabilitation care. These regions often struggle with clinician shortages, limited specialized services, and long travel distances, making it difficult for people in small, isolated communities to receive consistent, hands-on care.

I understand these struggles firsthand. I grew up in a small northern community in Canada with a total population of just 7,000 and very limited access to medical care. My family spent countless hours in the car, making the 16-hour round trip to see specialists a few times a year. I also knew many dentists who would fly into isolated towns in small propeller planes to reach communities where some residents had never had access to a dental exam before.

Virtual Care

The rise of virtual care has dramatically expanded access to healthcare. Telehealth, virtual rehab, and remote monitoring have become game-changers worldwide, bringing specialized care directly into people's homes.

Globally, countries like Australia are leading the way by embracing virtual rehabilitation platforms, such as **iAgeHealth**, alongside a national focus on telehealth, remote assessments, and robotic solutions to bridge care gaps.

In Canada's northern territories, mobile tech support and virtual health programs, such as the **Ontario Telemedicine Network (OTN)**, have helped overcome long-standing access issues.

Japan is piloting haptic robotics and virtual presence tools to address care shortages in rural regions, while India has rapidly expanded telehealth services, such as **eSanjeevani**, a national telemedicine platform, to reach remote villages.

Similarly, Brazil has made significant strides with **Telessaúde Brasil Redes**, bringing virtual consultations to underserved areas in the Amazon.

Together, these global efforts show how smart use of technology can break down distance barriers and deliver life-changing care to those who would otherwise be left out.

Haptic Robotics & Digital Assessments

Haptic robotics refers to robotic systems that simulate touch, pressure, and physical resistance, creating the sensation of guided, hands-on movement. These systems allow users to physically feel assistance or resistance during exercises, even when a therapist isn't present. This technology enables "hands-on" therapy to be delivered remotely, which provides an alternative for those who cannot easily travel for regular rehab appointments.

Rebless by H Robotics is a robotic-assisted therapy device designed for home use where a clinician will remotely guide the client to set up the device and provide supervision as it gently moves a patient's arm or leg through controlled ranges of motion. This allows for highly personalized, physically supported rehab, even from a distance.

In parallel, companies like **XRHealth** are offering in-home virtual reality (VR) therapy with insurance coverage, making remote rehab more accessible. Virtual robotic rehab care is already widely used in places like Korea, where remote robotic treatments are reimbursed at higher rates than traditional in-person sessions, accelerating the adoption of this technology.

When it comes to measuring movement without physical contact, camera-based platforms like **Kemtai** and **Orlando One** are excellent examples. These systems use computer vision and AI to track joint angles, body alignment, and exercise form, often capturing range of motion with more precision than the human eye.

This virtual assessment technology provides clinicians with real-time, objective data to monitor progress, correct form, and remotely coach patients.

C9 | Technology in the Home

The most interesting part of virtual care is that the client may actually get better care and more accurate assessments because these systems can track subtle joint movements frame by frame—details that are often difficult for the human eye to detect in a clinical setting.

Rehab robotics fall in two categories. The first includes robotic-assisted devices which physically move a patient's limb through controlled, therapeutic exercises. Bigger devices are usually deployed at a physical location, with smaller ones having more flexibility to be provided in the home environment with clinicians that can remotely monitor and adjust the treatment in real time. These robotics are usually working on only a specific joint or limb.

The second category involves whole body wearable exoskeleton systems like ones developed by **Cyberdyne, Human in Motion,** and **Wandercraft**. These provide powered support for walking, transfers, and mobility training and have significant impacts in spinal cord injuries, strokes and other life altering trauma by re-programming the brain through assisted motion. However, due to their high cost and the specialized expertise required to assist patients during use, these exoskeletons are still primarily only used in clinical settings. However, many are actively advancing toward a goal of safe, at-home use of them.

Together, haptic robotics, robotic-assisted therapy, wearable exoskeletons, and AI-powered assessments are transforming remote rehabilitation, making care more accessible, personalized, and often more precise than in-person methods.

Holograms and Virtual Presence: Expanding Access to Specialists in Rural Communities

The rise of hologram technology is creating powerful new ways to connect rural communities with specialized care. There are several hologram companies around the world that are transforming how we

Age in Place or Find a New Space

think about remote presence, especially for rural healthcare and virtual collaboration.

One of the most well-known is **Proto**, a U.S.-based company that developed life-sized hologram boxes to make real-time, face-to-face communication feel natural, even when people are separated by hundreds of miles. Proto's technology is already being used in hospitals, universities, and corporate settings to bring experts into the room instantly through holographic projection.

In the Netherlands, **Holoconnects** is creating similar experiences with their **Holobox**, a portable, freestanding hologram display that allows people to appear life-sized in real time. Holoconnects is actively working to bring this technology into virtual healthcare consults, education, and live events, making it easier for specialists to reach people in remote communities without ever needing to travel.

From Australia, **Voxon Photonics** is offering a different type of hologram experience with their **3D volumetric displays**. Unlike flat hologram boxes, Voxon's technology projects true three-dimensional images that can be viewed from any angle, like a hologram floating in space. This type of immersive display is gaining traction in healthcare simulation, training, and education, with exciting potential for hands-on remote therapy and patient demonstrations.

In Canada, **ARHT Media** is leading the way in holographic telepresence, particularly in the medical, corporate, and education sectors. Their **HoloPresence™** system has been used to bring specialists into conferences and classrooms as lifelike, real-time holograms, allowing for meaningful interaction across long distances.

Another emerging company is **IKIN**, based in the U.S., which focuses on portable, small-scale holographic displays. While IKIN's systems aren't life-sized, they offer an affordable, accessible way to incorporate 3D holograms into everyday communication and learning, with growing potential for healthcare applications.

So, how can holograms improve communication between patient and provider?

C9 | Technology in the Home

Consider the different ways that we communicate right now. An email can convey important information, but a phone call will ensure there are no misunderstandings. Zoom calls can add non-verbal context but it's still not quite the same as being in person.

The **U.S. Department of Veterans Affairs (VA)** use TVs installed in patient rooms so immobile patients can have face-to-face consults with specialists without needing to be moved.

Holograms differ in that they allow for an entire person to be projected, in color and in context, so that real-time, face-to-face conversations really start to feel like you are in person, even if you're hundreds of miles apart. Some hospitals even have this set up for patients so they can connect better with their families at home.

I see the potential benefit of how holograms could support rural health, having tried Proto Hologram at the Consumer Electronics Show a few years ago. I found it to be an ideal platform for patient and caregiver training because even though I'm being projected in a box, the experience is so realistic that I don't think it would matter.

From the box, I can demonstrate new exercises step-by-step and use the caregiver as an extension of my hands. For example, I can say, *"I want you to use your left hand to hold his arm up, just like you see me doing here,"* as I physically show the movement from my hologram box. I can see them return demonstrating my instructions and be able to provide real-time feedback.

This improves access to care tremendously by allowing patients to connect with specialists that they would not normally be able to see. In rural hospitals, these hologram units are being set up in dedicated virtual care rooms, where a local clinician can sit with the patient while a specialist appears "in the room" via hologram to review treatment plans, discuss lab results, and answer questions in a far more personal way than a traditional phone or video call.

Looking ahead, this same technology can be a supportive game-changer for rural physicians who may only encounter a rare case once a year. Alternatively, consider how supportive it would be to have a hologram in an operating room for a rural surgeon to consult with a specialist via hologram during a complex case.

The possibilities of technology are endless and I'm so excited to see how this technology will impact lives.

Intersection of Healthcare + Robotics

You've probably realized by now that I'm a total geek when it comes to robotics in the home. I still remember watching the adorable robot Baymax—"*I am your personal healthcare companion*"—in *Big Hero 6* with my kids, just a week before I was set to fly to Boston to give a talk at the **Toyota Research Institute** for their engineers.

It was almost surreal to think I'd soon be working on cutting-edge innovations just like in the movie. Even after years of collaborating with that team, it's all still so incredibly fun. One of the most rewarding outcomes from our long-term partnership was publishing our paper in *Applied Sciences* in January 2025, titled **"Exploring Embodiment Form Factors of a Home-Helper Robot: Perspectives from Care Receivers and Caregivers."**

In this study, we developed and evaluated three different designs for a home-helper robot, each aimed at assisting older adults with daily activities. What made this work so meaningful was that we didn't just build the robots—we deeply engaged with both caregivers and the people who would actually use them and created designs that were more user-friendly, practical, and genuinely aligned with real-world needs.

This past year, one of the visiting roboticists doing a summer internship at Toyota Research Institute came to a talk I gave about how clinicians use key points of control to safely and efficiently move patients, leveraging both biomechanical advantages and subtle tactile cues to guide motion. He and his colleague found this fascinating, and it was incredibly fun for me to share how clinicians actually work with patients in real life.

C9 | Technology in the Home

His lab went on to develop the **SPARCS** tool (*Structuring Physically Assistive Robotics for Caregiving with Stakeholders-in-the-loop*), which is a framework to help roboticists design real-world caregiving solutions by directly involving the people who will use them—caregivers, older adults, and occupational therapists. Once clinicians show how we perform a task like safely assisting a person out of bed or how a person moves in their daily routines, his team can break down the specific movements we use and then start programming the robot to perform those tasks.

This experience highlights the power of clinicians and engineers working together from the start. By combining clinical insight with engineering expertise, we co-create solutions that genuinely improve the quality of life for older adults. It's a great example of how the future of medicine is being shaped by interdisciplinary collaboration, where the best ideas come from listening, learning, and building together.

Future Application of Robotics

Imagine a future where someone with highly specialized skills, like an electrician, a plumber, or even a surgical specialist, could live in a major urban city and tap into your companion robot on your rural farm to help you with tasks you'd otherwise have no local access to. Your robot wouldn't just keep you company—it would become a bridge to expertise that would have been impossible to reach in the past.

One of my best friends, Mary Ellen, is a Da Vinci surgeon, and I've always been fascinated by the story of how that technology came to be. She was telling me that the Da Vinci robotic surgical system was originally developed by the **U.S. Department of Defense** with the idea that a surgeon could safely perform complex procedures remotely behind enemy lines, controlling a robot stationed in the field. It was about delivering expert care to soldiers in places where no surgeon could physically go, saving lives from a distance.

Age in Place or Find a New Space

Now, imagine applying that same concept to daily life. A skilled plumber in a different part of the city could remotely control your home robot to fix a leak in your kitchen. An electrician in another state could tap into your robot to safely rewire a faulty outlet. A specialist in one country could help repair an assistive device or mobility aid in another country. Your home wouldn't just be smart. It would be networked to a global pool of expertise, with robots acting as physical extensions of specialists around the world.

It's not as far off as it sounds. The foundational technology already exists. We've seen it in robot-assisted surgeries, remote-controlled machinery, and telepresence robotics. What's coming next is the blending of these technologies to create everyday solutions, where help is never out of reach, no matter where you live.

Mo-Go and Arteryxx: Smarter Mobility Through Collaboration

Mo-Go is a groundbreaking mobility solution, the world's first powered pant, designed to make moving easier, safer, and more natural for people who need extra support. Built right into clothing, Mo-Go provides discreet, wearable powered assistance that kicks in exactly when you need it—whether you're hiking uphill, walking longer distances, or just navigating everyday life. For older adults who want to stay active, independent, and confident without relying on bulky mobility aids, Mo-Go is the freedom you can wear.

Mo-Go's story is just as exciting as the technology itself. It started as a project at Google X and spun out into its own independent company, **Skip**, in 2023. The co-founders, Kathryn Zealand and Anna Roumiantseva, were personally driven by watching their loved ones' worlds shrink due to mobility challenges.

They wanted to build something that didn't just help people move, but helped them keep moving through life on their own terms. That's why

C9 | Technology in the Home

Skip partnered with **Arc'teryx's Advanced Concepts** team, experts in designing apparel for movement in tough environments, to bring Mo-Go to life. Together, they've created the world's first powered pant, designed with the real needs of real people at the center.

From Military Missions to Everyday Solutions

While the goal of this book is to provide practical, direct-to-consumer solutions that families can use right now, I always keep a close eye on emerging technologies, especially those coming from the worlds of space exploration, military development, and large-scale healthcare innovation hubs.

Historically, some of our most useful consumer products started in those arenas. Think about memory foam, which came from NASA, cordless vacuums inspired by drills used on the moon, and GPS, which was originally designed for military navigation. These high-tech solutions almost always start off as cost-prohibitive or specialized tools, but as they mature and scale, they often become more affordable and practical for everyday use.

I'll admit, it's also my inner MacGyver side that keeps me watching. I'm constantly thinking, *how can I recreate the same outcome with much cheaper components?* Even if the technology is still in the research and development phase, it's valuable to watch, because it shows us where the consumer market is headed.

When tracking what's coming next for home care, it's important to look upstream. Many of the consumer products we see in rehab, mobility, and smart home technology actually start in senior living communities, hospitals, and other specialized care settings. These are typically business-to-business (B2B) solutions where companies first test, refine, and validate their technologies before they trickle down to the consumer market. If you want to spot the next wave of home care innovations, pay attention to the senior living space—that's usually where

Age in Place or Find a New Space

new rehab technologies, fall prevention systems, and mobility aids first appear.

Some notable B2B solutions in the passive monitoring space are showing features that could be true game changers for aging in place. **Nami, Xander Kardian,** and **Pontosense** are developing ambient sensors that can passively monitor a home for subtle changes, like detecting when someone enters a room, falls, or is showing early signs of health changes that could lead to a fall.

For example, Xander Kardian's contactless health monitoring system is designed to track heart rate, breathing patterns, and even early signs of cardiac distress using radio frequency (RF) signals, offering continuous health monitoring without physical contact. Pontosense is also using radar-based sensing to passively detect changes in vital signs and behavior.

Meanwhile, **Magic Shield** is embedding vibration sensors directly into the floors to track gait, detect falls, and monitor movement patterns in a fully non-intrusive way.

We're also seeing powered robotic walkers like **Camino Robotics**, that can currently assist when walking up a hill but once combined with AI and cameras, has the ability to monitor gait and send alerts when step length shortens, or unsafe movement patterns emerge.

Predictive technology used in professional soccer to track ball trajectories is being investigated by **Sage Sentinel** to see if they can prevent a fall moments before it happens. It's a fascinating approach that I'm eager to see if it can be a disruptor in the space.

Following innovation hubs like the AgeTech Collaborative from AARP, AgeWell in Canada, and Lake Nona is a great way to stay up-to-date. Lake Nona is especially exciting because it's home to the VA's freestanding innovation center, SimVET, the UCF College of Medicine, and it's just a short distance from the Kennedy Space Center. Currently, Lake Nona is leading projects in smart homes, telepresence robotics, virtual rehabilitation, and precision healthcare, all of which are likely to reach the consumer level in the next few years.

That's where the future of home care is being built, long before it ever hits store shelves.

Technology Gives Independence

Having a plan isn't just reassuring for you. It's reassuring for everyone around you. I've seen it so many times: adult children start to panic when they can't reach their parent(s). The calls go unanswered, and suddenly they're jumping in the car, playing out worst-case scenarios during the 10-minute drive over, only to find their parent simply had the ringer off.

No one's happy in that situation. Your loved ones are stressed, and you're not getting the freedom and independence you want. This is where technology can really help. It gives you the freedom to live life on your own terms while offering quiet peace of mind to the people who care about you.

Now that you know the options and the possibilities for later, the next step is to think of this as part of your essential homework for building an aging-in-place plan.

Ask yourself:

- How will I get help if I fall?
- How can caregivers stay informed?
- What can I do to reduce social isolation?
- How can I make sure I'm managing my medications properly—especially pain or movement medications that work best when taken on a consistent schedule?
- How will I keep up with medical appointments or know when home health is scheduled to visit?
- How can I keep myself safe and secure at night? Are the doors locked? Is the garage door closed?

These aren't just checkboxes. They're key pieces of the puzzle that help you stay in control of your life and give your loved ones the confidence to support you without hovering.

Final Thoughts: The Future of the Home as a Care Partner

The future of independent living isn't just about adding smart devices. It's about transforming the home into an active care partner.

Smart insoles can help prevent wandering, sensors can detect subtle health changes and alert care teams, hydration reminders can be deployed, and systems that track sleep, social engagement, and daily patterns can catch early signs of decline.

Facial recognition can ensure secure access, predictive maintenance for appliances and cars reduce unexpected problems, and smart routines that lock doors and send safety alerts can make homes safer and more responsive. This is especially true for people with mobility challenges where voice-controlled locks, cameras, and appliances can return control and dignity to daily life.

These tools won't replace human caregivers, but they can help. A home can play the role of a vigilant care partner that spots abnormal trends and alerts human caregivers to take steps that only a human can take.

This future requires clinicians, engineers, caregivers, patients, and families to collaborate from the very beginning. By listening to each other, sharing real-world experiences, and co-designing solutions, we can create homes that don't just house people, they actively care for them.

I'm genuinely excited about what we can build together. ☺

C9 | Technology in the Home

Key Takeaways

- Most home-care technologies start in senior living and B2B spaces—watch innovation hubs like Lake Nona, AgeTech Collaborative, and Age-Well Canada to see what's coming next.
- Smart homes are becoming silent care partners, using ambient sensors and robotics to quietly monitor safety and detect subtle health changes without cameras or wearables.
- Start small with smart home tech, like using Amazon Alexa for lights or reminders, and gradually build from there at your own pace.
- Robotics like powered walkers and Labrador assistive carts now support everyday tasks, making movement, lifting, and carrying safer and easier at home.
- Virtual rehab, haptic robotics, and remote care are expanding access to therapy in rural and underserved areas, bringing expert care directly into the home.
- Voice assistants and smart home tools help people stay socially connected, mentally engaged, and emotionally supported through easy, hands-free technology.
- The future of fall prevention is passive and predictive, with smart sensors and AI quietly tracking movement patterns to detect risks before a fall happens.

Chapter Ten

Caregiving Relationships

Caregiving is an act of love and devotion, driven by a deep desire to keep our loved ones safe and recuperating at home. But caregiving can also feel like carrying the weight of the world.

In the United States, over 53 million individuals serve as unpaid family caregivers, providing essential support to loved ones with chronic illnesses, disabilities, or aging-related needs.

This care, valued at approximately $600 billion annually, underscores the critical role caregivers play in the healthcare system. If family caregivers stopped tomorrow, the formal healthcare system would collapse under the weight of the unmet need.

Caregivers are Superheroes

Caregivers don't start this journey thinking about themselves. They are doers. They are helpers. They see a need, and they pitch in to do what

C10 | Caregiving Relationships

they can. They are devoted family members who will do anything to help the person they love feel better. But sometimes, the balance and stability they offer comes at the expense of their own balance and stability.

Anyone with children knows exactly what I'm talking about. When your child is sick and crying from a raging fever, staying up all night to comfort them isn't a choice—it's simply part of the job description when you're caring for a little human you love deeply. But sacrificing a full night of sleep doesn't make it any easier to go to work the next day. The struggle to stay awake and concentrate while doing the job that provides for your family is tough. It's a difficult, exhausting balance.

Luckily, kids' immune systems mature, and they get better at not picking up every single bug that darkens the door of their school. They still get sick, but it's less work and life mostly goes back to normal in a few days' time.

In my experience, what sets caregiving for an older adult apart is its chronic, ongoing nature. At first, the caregiving needs might be short-term. Maybe they got Covid-19 and the hospitalization made them so weak that they need help to manage household chores for two or three weeks after they are discharged. Family, neighbors, and friends pitch in to help, and with time, they get their strength back and life goes back to normal.

But what happens when it's more serious? According to the **National Council on Aging**, fourteen million people, or one in four Americans age 65 and older, fall each year. The majority of the patients I saw in the home were due to fall-related injuries. A broken hip or femur bone was common. Falls on an outstretched arm (FOOSH) were also very common. Those generally resulted in fractured elbows, torn rotator cuff muscles, and dislocated shoulders. All of these take a lot of time to heal, as remodeling of bones doesn't begin until four to six weeks later.

The impact of a fall means that caregivers are needed to help suffering people get in and out of bed, transported by wheelchair to get to the bathroom, assisted to get on and off the toilet, manage toileting

Age in Place or Find a New Space

hygiene needs, transferred back into the wheelchair to then transfer into the shower, get bathed, dried off and dressed after. Every day. For many, many days.

But they, too, eventually get back to taking care of themselves and their homes, and life goes back to normal.

Exacerbations of chronic illnesses, such as chronic obstructive pulmonary disease, congestive heart failure, uncontrolled diabetes, or hypertension, often require hospitalization that can lead to weakness and deconditioning. In these cases, patients may not need as much help with self-care and recover more quickly, but chronic illnesses typically create caregiving needs that arise more frequently and require ongoing attention.

Progressive diseases like Parkinson's, Multiple Sclerosis, Alzheimer's, and some types of cancers have needs that can be very diverse in nature. Some will require periods of intense caregiving needs if they have an active progression. Some may only need supervision for safety if the disease is in a more stable phase.

Finally, traumatic injuries like spinal cord injuries, stroke, and amputation can have significant needs for months or years following the injuries. They need help with managing self-care, care of the home, assistance with their home exercise programs, transport to multiple appointments, and hopefully, transport to community engagement activities like attending church services, social exercise groups, support groups, and book clubs. Some will recover more than others depending on age, severity, and location of the injury, but in almost all cases, there will be a lifelong need for some level of assistance as they navigate a new normal.

The most critical thing to understand is that family caregivers are often juggling all of these responsibilities while also holding down a job to cover the growing expenses. Some families are fortunate enough to have relatives who can share the load, but many live far apart, making coordination a logistical nightmare. It can be incredibly challenging to manage who is arriving, who is leaving, and whether someone will be available to take their loved one to an important medical appointment.

C10 | Caregiving Relationships

Given what I've just shared, I'm sure you can understand why I often feel that the caregivers look worse than the patients do. And that's not just my opinion. AARP's Caregiving in the U.S. report paints a stark picture. About 40 percent of family caregivers report high levels of emotional stress. More than one in five caregivers report feeling alone in their role. Financial stress is another common thread—caregivers often cut back on paid work, reduce hours, or even leave jobs entirely to meet caregiving demands. This can devastate their own retirement savings and financial security.

Worse, caregiver stress isn't just emotional—it's physical. Studies show that over half of caregivers suffer from lower back pain and musculoskeletal injuries, especially when assisting with daily transfers. The risks multiply for caregivers supporting individuals with neurodegenerative diseases like Parkinson's or dementia, where the need for help can continue for years.

Chronic sleep loss, social withdrawal, depression, and anxiety are common among caregivers. But what options do they have? If they don't have a support system, they can't leave their spouse alone. And if there isn't money for respite care, what choice do they have but to soldier on, ignoring their own needs? It's a rock and a hard place.

Why Caregivers Matter

Caregivers are not optional background supporters. They are lifelines. Without them, many older adults would have no choice but to get care in a congregate living environment. The presence of caregivers is what makes it even possible to recover at home or age in place. They are vital, and this is why I care so much.

Occupational therapists are usually ordered when a patient has a specific need. An illness or injury has created a difference between who they were before the incident and what they are able to do after. Our job is to assess what their previous level of function (PLOF) was, assess what their current level of function (CLOF) is, and figure out what interventions are needed to make those match again.

As you can imagine, when a person has just arrived home from the hospital, their caregiving needs are significant. That's why, in the first few visits, my top priority is providing caregiver training for safe transfers. I often remind families, "If the caregiver is exhausted or has tweaked their back during this morning's transfer, how will the patient manage on their own?" The answer is, they can't. When a caregiver is injured, the ripple effect is profound. In my opinion, supporting caregivers is not a luxury, it's a necessity. That's why I see my role as supporting both the patient and the caregiver in equal measure. One cannot survive without the other.

The Challenges of Caregiving

Being a caregiver has many difficulties that they face on a daily basis. Activities like lifting, transferring, and assisting with bathing carry a high risk of injury when done without training.

There is a significant cognitive burden involved in simply keeping up with all the visiting clinicians, follow-up appointments, and daily medications that need to be managed.

On top of that, there are the emotional challenges—watching your loved one decline or trying to navigate the shifting relationship dynamics as roles change from husband and wife to patient and caregiver.

Once you add in the financial challenges of covering medical equipment, home modifications, and sometimes lost wages, the stress can be overwhelming.

But the part that I worry most about is the profound isolation that caregivers report. Days get filled up quickly with appointments, medications, and checklists. Social activities get skipped, and without scheduled meet-ups, friendships drift and phone calls cease.

C10 | Caregiving Relationships

You Have an Army: AARP's Toolbox for Caregivers

AARP has created one of the most comprehensive caregiver support hubs in the country, filled with practical, accessible resources designed to help you survive, and thrive, on this journey.

The AARP website has a **Caregiving Resource Center** with lots of great resources, such as:

- **Step-by-Step Guides**: If you're getting ready for a loved one to come home from the hospital or trying to figure out long-term care plans, AARP's caregiving guides break things down in simple, practical steps so you know what to expect and how to get prepared.
- **Financial Workbooks**: These help you track caregiving expenses, understand long-term care costs, and plan proactively using AARP's Long-Term Care Calculator.
- **Legal Tools**: AARP offers guidance on essential documents like power of attorney, healthcare proxies, and setting up wills and trusts.
- **Community Connections**: Through the AARP caregiving forums and Facebook Live events, you can connect with other caregivers, ask questions, and get real-time support. Caregivers who join these communities often say that hearing "me too" from others lifts the weight of isolation.
- **Quick Self-Care Strategies**: AARP offers 15-minute self-care ideas—things like a quiet cup of tea, breathing exercises, or short walks that can make a real difference.

AARP HomeFit Guide & HomeFit App

The AARP HomeFit Guide and AARP HomeFit App are practical, user-friendly resources designed to help people of all ages make their homes safer, more comfortable, and better suited for aging in place.

The **HomeFit Guide** offers step-by-step checklists, room-by-room safety recommendations, and simple home modification ideas to improve accessibility, many of which can be done affordably or as DIY projects.

The companion **HomeFit App** makes this process interactive, allowing users to virtually walk through a home, identify potential hazards, and explore personalized solutions right from their smartphone or tablet.

The guide and app empower individuals and caregivers to create living spaces that support independence, prevent falls, and adapt as needs change over time. These are free resources that you can order paper copies of or download from their website.

"Conversations for the Future: Finances, Health, and Housing" is a webinar I co-hosted with AARP's Caregiving Expert, Amy Goyer, and AARP's Legal Expert, Amanda Singleton, back in November 2022. In it, we discuss what to expect and what you need to plan for: covering home modifications, caregiving considerations, and key legal preparations. At the time of this book's publication, the webinar is still available to watch on the AARP Programs Facebook page.

Tips to Protect Your Body and Sanity

As an occupational therapist, I've spent years in the homes of family caregivers. Here's what I teach my caregivers:

- **Safe Transfers**: When helping someone from sitting to standing, cue them: "Nose over toes, then lift." Focus on weight shifting. Use friction-reducing sheets like **Comfort Linen** to reposition in bed without lifting.

C10 | Caregiving Relationships

- **Use Assistive Devices**: Don't wait for a crisis to install grab bars or purchase a tub transfer bench. Make sure you have a chair with arms that they can push themselves up from to avoid your pulling on them. Tools don't just help the patient. They decrease the physical strain on a caregiver and help a caregiver anticipate what the next step will be.
- **Practice Energy Conservation**: Break tasks into manageable pieces throughout the day. Have patients sit while grooming or dressing so that you work at your optimal biomechanical range, which is between your shoulders and your knees. Engage your core when moving someone and remember to breathe.
- **Don't "Steal their Therapy:"** Your job isn't to do everything. It's to show them what you want them to do, give them encouragement with verbal cues or hand-over-hand cues. Don't take over, let them try. This builds their strength and protects yours.
- **Invest in Respite Care**: Even a few hours a week can be transformative. Call your local Area Agency on Aging to find out what resources they have available to help you. **Care Yaya** hires local college kids in medical professions to help at a lower cost. The bonus is all the young energy that makes older adults smile and gives you a reason to smile, too.
- **Lean on Technology**: Use tools like Alexa for medication and appointment reminders, social robots like **ElliQ**, and passive monitoring like **Envoy at Home** or **Caregiver Smart Solutions**, which can send alerts to long-distance caregivers. It's important to note that these technologies do not connect to emergency services but instead use discreet sensor technology to detect motion in the home in a non-intrusive way.
- **Plan Financially**: Use AARP's long-term care calculators and workbooks to prepare for the cost of caregiving. Planning reduces crisis decision-making and guilt.

How to Stay Connected

Social connection and access to healthcare are lifelines. With basic tools like FaceTime, Alexa, and Zoom, older adults can attend virtual classes, connect with loved ones, or have telehealth appointments.

But tech goes further than that. **OnScreen** connects with a person's TV and allows caregivers to "drop in" visually without needing a tech-savvy parent to push buttons. **Loop Village** offers older adults an easy, engaging way to participate in virtual group activities and can be connected with OnScreen.

To move a relationship back to husband and wife, I love interactive, live-streamed travel experiences with **Discover.Live** or **Wowzitude.** Many families have enjoyed doing the ancestry tours that can include many members on the Zoom platform at once and be able to talk to the local guides directly to ask questions.

I love combining exercise with travel, and the **Bike Labyrinth** app takes that a step further by allowing users and their loved ones to virtually pedal through cities they've visited together in the past. It also offers fun experiences like sled dog tours and leisurely walks through the tulip gardens in the Netherlands.

The **Color-Coded Chef** was built for individuals with cognitive challenges and has color-coded tools with pictogram step-by-step instructions. I love this as a great shared experience for grandkids and grandparents to connect over cooking a meal together in the kitchen.

What about for the patient? **Whispp** transforms speech for those with vocal impairments by recording the patient's healthy voice and enabling them to communicate directly with family for more independent and meaningful conversations. This eliminates the need for a caregiver to assist.

How to Preserve Modesty and Dignity

One of the biggest unspoken challenges in caregiving, especially in father-daughter or mother-son dynamics, is how to help with personal

C10 | Caregiving Relationships

care while preserving modesty. Bathing, dressing, and toileting are intimate tasks and, for many, emotionally complex.

In my work, it's all about planning ahead. I often have the patient change into an oversized T-shirt, depending on their functional level, and guide the caregiver on how to assist with a safe transfer to the shower. We make sure the water is already set to the preferred temperature, the shower hose is within easy reach with the pause button engaged, and all bathing supplies, including a long-handled bathing sponge, are nearby—either in a basket or on a shampoo shelf grab bar. The shower curtain is drawn for privacy. When ready, the patient removes the T-shirt and hands it to the caregiver, who remains just outside the shower, chatting with them to provide reassurance and ensure they feel safe throughout the process.

When bathing is finished, the caregiver hands the patient a towel to dry off as much as possible, then passes them the oversized T-shirt to put back on. The caregiver drapes a towel over the seat and backrest of the wheelchair so that when the patient sits down, the towel can absorb the remaining water from the back and between the legs. Caregivers are usually comfortable drying the legs, or I'll have them use a bathrobe or large towel to cover the front of the legs. Because of the length, patients can often tuck it under their thighs, and when they go to cross their legs, the lower legs make contact and can dry off that way.

I recognize this is a lot of work, but once people have done it a few times, it becomes a well-orchestrated ballet. I'm sure there are other workarounds that other OTs have developed, but this is the best system I've found that works for the majority of mother-son and father-daughter caregiving situations.

There are a couple of commercial solutions that could also be good options. One of my favorites is the **Blue Hug** which is modesty gown made of a neoprene shell with long bi-directional zippers along the front and sides. The wetsuit material helps keep the patient warm, the sensation of the water provides a calming, weighted-blanket effect, and the zippers allow easy access to bathe one area at a time while keeping the rest of the body covered.

They have had a lot of success with using this modesty gown for clients with dementia who may not recognize a caregiver and understandably, be unwilling to get undressed to take a shower with them in the room.

This is also a great solution for older adults who have just moved into a community setting and need help with bathing. Having a garment helps to reduce the discomfort and awkwardness of being bathed by someone they don't yet know.

Final Thoughts: You Are Not Alone in This Journey

Caregiving is one of the hardest and most beautiful acts of love you will ever give. It can feel heavy, exhausting, and at times, completely overwhelming—but it is also meaningful, life-changing work that allows our loved ones to heal, thrive, and stay home. I hope this chapter has not only validated your experience but also provided you with real, actionable strategies and resources to lighten your load.

You don't have to do this alone. There is a growing network of tools, communities, and people who are here to walk alongside you—people who understand what you're facing.

My deepest wish is that you feel empowered to ask for help, to take small steps to protect your own well-being, and to remember that your health matters too. You are not just a caregiver. You are a lifeline. Your work has incredible value, and when we support caregivers, we build stronger, healthier families and communities.

C10 | Caregiving Relationships

Key Takeaways

- While caregiving is a selfless act of love and devotion, caregivers still need to take time away to care for themselves.
- Call in help when it makes sense; doing it all leads to burnout.
- Caregiver stress is not just emotional but also presents itself physically.
- Social connection and access to health care are lifelines.
- Do what you can to preserve the patient's dignity.

Chapter Eleven

Age in Place or Find a New Space®

Deciding to age in place is a lot like planning a vacation. You don't just wake up one morning and hop on a plane. First, there's the decision: *Are we doing this?* Then you check your bank account—what's the budget? After that, you start dreaming: beach or mountains? Cruise or cabin? You narrow it down based on what kind of experience you're really looking for. And of course, you build in a few backup plans, because we all know not everything goes according to the itinerary.

Planning to age in place works the same way. It begins with a choice, followed by a reality check, a bit of dreaming, and a great deal of thoughtful planning.

I created **Age in Place or Find a New Space®** to guide clients through the mental exercise of planning ahead so they'd have options ready to go if life took an unexpected turn.

One couple had lived in their three-storey home for over thirty years and just couldn't imagine leaving it. But once we walked through the renovation plans, the cost to reconfigure the stairs, add a main-floor

C11 | Age in Place or Find a New Space®

bedroom and bathroom, and widen the doorways was much more than the cost of buying a different house that would require less work. For them, it wasn't just about money; it was about the stress of living through months of construction and realizing that the layout still might not fully meet their future needs.

Another client had her heart set on retrofitting her historic home, only to discover that zoning restrictions and structural limitations would prevent the changes she needed. In both cases, exploring alternate housing options was an opportunity to reimagine what safety, comfort, and freedom could look like with a blank slate.

In using my vacation metaphor, what happens when you have your heart set on a specific location, only to discover that an international festival is in town and the hotel rooms have been booked solid for a month already? You could work to find alternative ways to make it work like staying in a town nearby with the added expense of needing to rent a car or if it was important to you to stay in the city, you could forgo the comfort of a hotel room and try your luck with a vacation rental or a campground. You might also decide that it's not worth the hassle and opt for an alternative location.

It's the same with housing. You can absolutely *try* to make your original plan work, but it may come with added costs, compromises, and new logistics you didn't anticipate. Maybe you rent equipment, bring in outside help, or adjust your expectations. And sometimes, after weighing all that, you realize: this plan no longer fits the vision you had.

That's not failure. That's wisdom.

When we let go of a rigid picture of how things are "supposed to be," we make space for something better—something that supports your life as it is now, not as it once was or as you hoped it might be. That could mean finding a home all on one level, moving closer to family, or choosing a community with built-in support. No matter the result, the mindset shift is the important part. It's not about giving up. It's about choosing what serves you best.

Age in Place or Find a New Space

Make Decisions Based on Your Values

So, what do you do with the realization that your original plan may no longer be the best fit?

My advice? Always go back to your non-negotiables.

For many people, one of the most important factors isn't the structure of the home at all, it's the community around it. If you love your neighbors, have deep roots in your area, or rely on a trusted network of friends, healthcare providers, or faith communities, then staying close by may matter more than staying in your exact house. And that's okay. In fact, that clarity is powerful.

Instead of forcing your current home to work, try this: start going to open houses in your neighborhood. Explore other options that are already available to you. Walk through those homes through the eyes of an occupational therapist. Look at the width of doorways, the layout of bathrooms, the number of steps, and the location of the laundry. Think about what it would take to live there comfortably—not just today, but in five or ten years.

If the modifications you'd need in a new home are similar to what your current home requires, you may be able to use your recent contractor quotes as a baseline to estimate the cost. This is where a great local real estate agent becomes a true partner. A knowledgeable agent knows what's available in your area and, more importantly, they often have trusted contractor connections who can give you a ballpark estimate for potential modifications.

This approach gives you a clearer financial picture. Instead of comparing the list price of a new home to your current situation, you're comparing the total cost of staying versus moving, with all the work factored in. That "cheaper" house down the street? It might come with extensive renovations that push the final cost well above what you expected. Meanwhile, another home, maybe with a little more upfront cost, could already have the bones and layout you need, saving you time, money, and stress down the line. It's so important to keep the big picture in mind and not be tempted to automatically choose the cheapest option.

C11 | Age in Place or Find a New Space®

It's about choosing the right one for *you* based on your priorities, your health, and your long-term comfort.

A helpful tool for easily comparing neighborhoods across the United States is AARP's Livability Index.

Created by AARP's Housing and Livable Communities leaders, Rodney Harrell and Shannon Guzman, this data-driven tool evaluates neighborhoods in seven key categories that influence quality of life, especially for older adults who want to age in place.

The **Livability Index** provides an easy-to-understand numerical score (0–100) to help people easily compare locations. It empowers individuals to choose communities that offer safety, accessibility, affordability, and meaningful social engagement, making aging at home safer, more connected, and more fulfilling. The index evaluates neighborhoods based on housing, transportation, environment, health, engagement, opportunity, and neighborhood access.

What to Look for at an Open House: Through OT Eyes

Now that you're well-versed in what to look for, I want you to practice bringing your OT mindset with you when you go to your first open house. Here's what you to pay special attention to:

Entry & Exterior

- Is there at least one step-free entrance?
- Are walkways wide, well-lit, and in good condition?
- Could a ramp be added without major excavation?
- Is the driveway flat or sloped?

Age in Place or Find a New Space

Hallways & Doorways

- Are doorways at least 32 inches wide (preferably 36 inches) to accommodate walkers or wheelchairs?
- Can hallways comfortably accommodate two people walking side-by-side?
- Are there tight turns or pinch points that could become a barrier later?

Bathrooms

- Is there at least one bathroom with enough floor space to maneuver?
- Is the shower curbless, or could it be converted?
- Are there existing grab bars or places where blocking could be added for future grab bar installation?
- Is there room for a shower chair or caregiver assistance, if needed?

Kitchen & Laundry

- Are commonly used items reachable without a stepstool?
- Is there room to work seated or standing, with clear access to appliances?
- Are washer/dryer units front-loading and easily accessible?
- Could pull-out shelving or task lighting be added?

General Layout

- Are essential rooms on one level (bedroom, full bathroom, kitchen)?
- Is there a logical flow between rooms, or lots of unnecessary backtracking and sharp turns?
- Does the lighting feel bright and even, with minimal glare and shadows?

C11 | Age in Place or Find a New Space®

Case Study #1: We're Not Leaving Our Neighborhood!

One of my favorite stories comes from a couple who had lived in their two-storey home for decades and were adamant about aging in place. But when we walked through the cost of modifying the stairs, creating a main-floor suite, and widening narrow doorways, the number was staggering. Still, they didn't want to leave their neighborhood.

So, they started attending open houses within a one-mile radius, just to see.

A few weekends in, they found a charming one-storey home with a wide hallway, a zero-step entry from the garage, and a spacious primary bathroom that needed only a few small tweaks. With the renovation estimate from their contractor in hand, we compared costs, and to their surprise, the new home won out by a long shot. Best of all, they stayed in their community, near their friends and doctors. The move gave them peace of mind, and the process gave them control over their decision, not panic.

Case Study #2: Do the Homework, Find the Peace

Another couple I worked with thought they were ready to dive straight into renovations. They'd lived in their home for decades and loved it, so they knew they were willing to invest in it. However, the minute they opened the email and saw the first contractor's quote, everything came to a screeching halt. The cost was double what I typically see in bigger cities. Of course, their first reaction was, "Carol, are we being taken advantage of?"

Thankfully, the answer was "no." The reality is that they lived in a small-to-medium-sized city where the price quoted was simply what the local market would bear. We did our due diligence, reaching out to five other contractors, but every proposal came back within a few thousand

Age in Place or Find a New Space

dollars of each other. No one was overcharging. It was just the economic reality.

If you dig a little deeper, you'll understand why. In bigger cities, there's a much larger labor pool to draw from. Skilled tradespeople often reside in surrounding suburbs, and the high volume of available workers drives down prices. But in smaller cities, the supply is thinner, and when you're hiring for quality, you're going to pay for it.

Fortunately, this couple wasn't in crisis mode. They had the gift of time as a proactive couple, and they used it wisely. Instead of rushing forward, we decided on a plan to spend six months fully exploring their options. They toured homes within a one-mile radius, then expanded their search to other parts of the city. They even considered relocating closer to their daughter in another state.

Our approach was methodical. I had them create a binder and spreadsheet, tracking costs, layouts, condition of homes, and features. Nothing was off the table. They took this mission very seriously. They visited open houses. They explored 55+ communities. They toured continuing care retirement communities (CCRCs) both locally and near their daughter. And what they discovered surprised them.

Yes, some of the newer 55+ communities had lower upfront costs, but they came with significantly smaller square footage, which was a dealbreaker. Other homes in their neighborhood? They had similar layout challenges to their own, meaning renovation costs would have been comparable. And the all-in pricing for CCRCs? Nearly identical to the cost of modifying their existing home.

So, what did they decide?

They came back to the decision table with fresh eyes, realistic expectations, and a deep sense of clarity and chose to move forward with the original home renovation plan.

The difference? They understood the numbers.

What once felt like sticker shock had become a well-researched, intentional investment. Now, whenever they step into that bathroom, they see thoughtful planning and smart choices—and they feel good about the money they spent. Because in the end, all that research and reflection led them to one clear truth: there's no place like home.

Case Study #3: Downsizing Isn't for Everyone

One of the core goals I encourage my clients to consider when aging in place is finding ways to reduce the maintenance demands of their home. Not because I want to eliminate all physical work—quite the opposite.

In fact, activities like gardening, housework, and light yard maintenance can offer tremendous benefits: they provide a sense of purpose, keep the body moving, and maintain routines.

This aligns with the characteristics found in Blue Zones—the regions of the world where people live the longest, healthiest lives. In these communities, daily movement is integrated into life, not through structured workouts, but through meaningful, routine activities such as walking, cooking, and tending to gardens. (See Box 2 for more information.)

But here's where it gets nuanced.

Downsizing for me isn't about doing less. It's about prioritizing doing what's important. When clients downsize intentionally, they free up time and energy that would otherwise be drained by constant upkeep. If your daily routine is so consumed by cleaning, home repairs, and maintenance tasks that it eats up 75 percent of your energy reserves, it doesn't leave much room for the parts of life that truly fill your cup like playing with grandkids, enjoying your hobbies, or just being present with loved ones.

In those moments, the home that once symbolized independence and comfort can start to feel more like a burden or even a prison. Downsizing offers a way out, not necessarily out of your neighborhood or community, but out of the time drain. It's an aging-in-place strategy that prioritizes your values: less time fixing, more time enjoying.

Age in Place or Find a New Space

What Are *Blue Zones*—and What Do They Teach Us About Home?

Blue Zones are five regions around the world where people consistently live the longest, healthiest lives:

> Okinawa, Japan
> Sardinia, Italy
> Nicoya, Costa Rica
> Ikaria, Greece
> Loma Linda, California

What do these places have in common? Their residents don't live longer because of fancy supplements or home gyms. They thrive because their daily lives naturally support movement, connection, and a sense of purpose. People in Blue Zones:

-- Move regularly by walking, gardening, or doing chores

-- Maintain strong ties with family and community

-- Have a sense of purpose ("Ikigai" in Japan, "Plan de Vida" in Costa Rica)

-- Live in environments that make the healthy choice the easy one

So, what does this mean for aging in place? It means the goal isn't to eliminate activity, it's to create a lifestyle where meaningful movement and human connection happen naturally.

Downsizing is a way to get closer to that. A smaller, well-designed home with lower upkeep gives you back the time and energy to live more like the people in Blue Zones—spending your days doing the things that keep you grounded, joyful, and well.

Box 2

C11 | Age in Place or Find a New Space®

Of course, this isn't the right path for everyone. But I bring it up with clients because it reframes the conversation. Downsizing isn't about giving something up; it's about scaling your environment to fit your life today, not the one you lived twenty years ago.

That said, we also need to have an honest conversation about expectations, because downsizing has been romanticized. It's easy to watch a fun reality TV show about tiny home living and think, "That's the dream—minimal stuff, more freedom, and a cuter kitchen." But those shows are carefully scripted and styled to create that illusion.

I always tell my clients: If I took a laundry basket and cleared off every inch of my kitchen counters, mine would look huge, too. What you're seeing on TV isn't real life. It's a highlight reel. And when it comes to living in a significantly smaller space, real life has a lot more laundry, clutter, and elbow-bumping than what makes the final cut.

That's why I encourage people to look past the fantasy and get curious about what downsizing really feels like in practice. Because once the excitement wears off, you're left with the logistics, the emotions, and the everyday realities of a new lifestyle.

Take, for example, the couple I worked with. When they first began thinking about downsizing, they found themselves caught between excitement and anxiety. Their two-storey colonial had served them well for over 35 years. It was filled with memories—and a lot of stuff. But with their kids grown and the stairs becoming more noticeable with each passing year, they started to wonder: Could a smaller home make life easier?

They took the next few months to really *live* into the idea. They limited themselves to just the downstairs of their current home to see how it felt to live with less space. They started purging items room by room, hiring a professional organizer to help them sort through years of accumulated belongings, including boxes of their adult kids' high school trophies and childhood artwork.

They also got very honest with themselves. They realized they still loved to host their grandchildren for sleepovers and holiday dinners.

A one-bedroom condo wasn't going to cut it. But a smaller home *with* a dedicated guest room? That could work. Their new goal shifted: they weren't just looking to shrink, they were looking to right-size.

Eventually, they found a ranch-style home in a nearby neighborhood with wide hallways, a manageable yard, and just enough space to live comfortably without the burden of constant upkeep. It had good bones, and with a few small modifications, it would support them well into the future.

The outcome? They moved, but not in a rush. They did it on their timeline, with clarity and confidence. They had fewer rooms, but more functionality. Less clutter, but more peace. And best of all, they had a home that was aligned with the life they *actually* wanted to live.

Case Study #4: When It's Time to Pivot

For some, the idea of a retirement community sparks anxiety. They imagine giving up freedom, routines, or the comfort of a home they've known for decades. But here's what I've learned: Aging in place can work beautifully, but it often requires piecing together layers of support including managing caregivers, coordinating home repairs, scheduling transportation. For some people, that patchwork solution works great. For others, it becomes exhausting, especially when cognitive changes, complex medical needs, or social isolation come into play.

That's when the conversation shifts from "Can I stay here?" to "Would another setting help me live more fully?" One of my clients was a couple in their mid-80s. They had lived independently for years, managing just fine with a bit of help here and there with grocery delivery, house cleaning, a friendly neighbor to take out the trash. But after Mr. J.'s Parkinson's symptoms progressed, and a few minor falls turned into a serious hospitalization, everything changed. Mrs. J., still sharp and fiercely independent in her 80s, was now managing medication schedules, personal care, and a husband who occasionally forgot where he was in the house. The mental load was taking its toll.

C11 | Age in Place or Find a New Space®

Their adult children were worried. They lived out of state and were calling constantly to check in, coordinate services, and manage crises from afar. Everyone was trying to make aging in place work, but it was becoming harder to ignore the signs of burnout, both emotional and physical.

So, we got real. We talked about the quality of life, for both of them. They had worked hard all their life, saved everything to put their kids through school, and it was hard for their kids to see them struggling. They felt helpless and didn't know how to approach the subject without sounding like they were trying to tell them what to do.

On the side of my clients, they didn't want to feel like they were "giving up," and I assured them they weren't. There was no golden trophy handed out for enduring hardships because they *thought* that was what was expected of them. Understanding that exploring other options didn't equate to failure helped them see how what they were doing was not needed. When they were able to put down the burden they were carrying around, they got flexibility in return.

I got them connected with a local assisted living locator, a professional who helps older adults and families find senior living communities that match their care needs, lifestyle, and budget, usually at no cost to the client. They toured a few independent and assisted living communities with that professional, just to gather information and see what it was like.

One of them just felt right as soon as they walked through the doors. It wasn't sterile or stuffy; it was warm, modern, and filled with natural light. The apartments were private and familiar, but with just enough built-in support to make daily life more manageable. There was a dining room, scheduled transportation, and most importantly, a medication management program that gave Mrs. J. some much-needed relief.

The decision wasn't easy. It was more than they had planned to spend. But it lifted the weight she'd been carrying alone. For the first time in a long time, she didn't have to do everything or be everything. She had help now, and that changed everything.

They moved into a small, thoughtfully designed unit just 10 minutes from their old neighborhood. Within weeks, Mrs. J. was sleeping better. She started attending a morning chair yoga class. Mr. J. joined a men's discussion group. Their kids stopped calling every hour to check in. The whole family exhaled.

The outcome? They didn't feel like they had lost their independence. They felt like they had regained their lives.

Final Thoughts

Like so many times in your life, deciding where your next chapter lies is a stepwise journey. That next space might be your current home, a better-sized home in your neighborhood, or a fresh start in a retirement community. There's no single "right" answer—only the one that fits *you* best right now.

It can be easy to get stuck in analysis paralysis, just like when you're weighing grab bar decisions or debating the logistics of a full bathroom remodel. But here's the gentle reminder I offer to my clients: you're allowed to try something, learn from it, and change your mind.

That's not failure, that's growth.

When you take the pressure off needing a perfect solution and instead give yourself permission to explore, it creates space for calm, curiosity, and clarity. You've done it before—made a decision, changed your mind, and kept going.

This is no different. So, give yourself grace. Take stock of your options. Be honest about what you value. And know that your first choice doesn't have to be your final one. Maybe the first move isn't perfect, but the experience gets you closer to what will be a better fit. And remember, the goal isn't perfection. It's alignment. The most important choice you can make is this: to live in a space that supports the life you want to keep living now, and in the years to come.

C11 | Age in Place or Find a New Space®

Key Takeaways

- The best living arrangement is the one that fits your current needs and lifestyle.
- Start with your values and non-negotiables before making any housing decision.
- Explore your options early so you can plan from a place of confidence, not crisis.
- Use cost estimates as information—not roadblocks—to guide informed choices.
- Downsizing works best when it frees up time and energy for what truly matters.
- Retirement communities aren't for everyone, but they can offer structure and support.
- You're allowed to change your mind—this journey is about flexibility, not perfection.

Chapter Twelve

Aging in Place with Parkinson's Disease

You might be wondering why I've included a chapter on Parkinson's Disease in a book about aging in place. The truth is, if you haven't met someone living with Parkinson's yet, you likely will. Parkinson's Disease (PD) is now the second-fastest-growing neurological condition in the world. It affects nearly 10 million people globally, and diagnosis rates are expected to double in the coming decades, largely due to people living longer. The longer we live, the higher the likelihood of developing Parkinson's.

Empathy begins with understanding, not just the clinical facts. My hope is to demystify the disease and equip professionals working with older adults with a foundational understanding of what Parkinson's is, how it progresses, and what can be done to maintain quality of life.

When clients or their family members receive this diagnosis, it's often shocking and deeply unsettling. In that moment, it means everything to know that even the non-clinical members of their team—financial advisors, interior designers, architects—understand what they're up against. It brings tremendous comfort to know that those they know, like and trust are prepared, empathetic, and ready to adapt their expertise through the lens of this new reality.

My Journey with Parkinson's Disease

"By any chance, is her name Carol?" It was 2008 at **Brooks Rehabilitation** in Jacksonville, Florida, and that unexpected question marked the beginning of a powerful reconnection. The person asking was Melanie Bassett Lomaglio—physical therapist, professor at the **University of St. Augustine**, neuro-residency mentor to my PT partner, Kathy Mannion, and a student-athlete whom I knew from my college years.

This is a story about how the universe quietly places the right people in your life, sometimes long before you realize you need them.

I had joined the incredible team at Brooks Inpatient Rehabilitation Hospital in 2006, where occupational therapy manager Alice Krauss and physical therapy manager Donni Welch-Rawls led with purpose and vision. At that time, Brooks was the only inpatient rehabilitation hospital in Northeast Florida, and our first-floor gym was a dynamic space where occupational therapists and physical therapists worked side by side. We treated everything from spinal cord injuries and strokes to amputations and complex orthopedic cases, all grounded in the latest evidence-based care.

Brooks Rehabilitation has always been rooted in both compassion and innovation. Nearly 20 years ago, we were already using robotics to help stroke survivors with hemiplegia regain function — something that's only become more common in rehabilitation settings in recent years. Today, Brooks Rehabilitation has grown into a comprehensive health system with multiple inpatient rehabilitation hospitals and a new facility underway in partnership with the **Mayo Clinic** in Arizona. I now collaborate with Brooks Rehabilitation through their **Center of**

Age in Place or Find a New Space

Innovation, helping to validate technologies that can elevate patient care and transform outcomes.

However, the roots of this story extend even further back to Montreal, Canada.

McGill University, often referred to as the "Harvard of Canada," was where I spent my college years. As a member of the varsity swim team, I trained 20–30 hours a week, in addition to my full-time studies. The track coach's office was next to our pool, and when one of his runners got injured, he'd send them to train with us in the water. That's how I met Melanie Lomaglio 29 years ago.

After graduation, we lost touch. And then one day, by complete coincidence, she sat at my empty desk at Brooks. She noticed my picture and recognized me. Somehow, all these years later, we had both ended up marrying Americans and were only living forty-five minutes apart in North Florida.

When we finally had a chance to catch up, I learned that Melanie had devoted her career to treating people with Parkinson's and related neurological conditions. She and her husband, David, also a physical therapist, had opened several clinics in St. Augustine, including a dedicated Parkinson's and Neurologic Health Center. At the time, I knew very little about Parkinson's. But that would soon change.

Years later, I got a call from my mother-in-law. She and my father-in-law had just returned from the neurologist. Ted had been diagnosed with Parkinson's Disease. I felt heartbroken. Up to that point, my experience as an occupational therapist had shown me how little impact traditional therapy seemed to have on progressive diseases like Parkinson's. I didn't know what to do, but I knew who to call.

Melanie was upbeat and hopeful. She told me about the evolving approach to Parkinson's care—specifically, the power of targeted exercise to slow progression and improve quality of life. She encouraged us to schedule an appointment right away.

That visit inspired me to learn more. Melanie's optimism, deep knowledge, and practical strategies opened a door I didn't know existed.

C12 | Aging in Place with Parkinson's Disease

Before we even left her clinic, I had already registered for the next **Parkinson's Wellness Recovery (PWR!)** certification course. I earned my certification a few months later and felt energized to have such a powerful new tool in my toolbox.

After the course, I put my newfound skills (with a little MacGyver spirit) to work. I began using the movement patterns with all my patients, not just those with Parkinson's disease, curious to see what might happen. The results were remarkable.

One of my most memorable cases was a man who had lived with chronic back pain for three decades. Nothing had worked, not surgery, not injections. But with modified PWR! exercises, he became pain-free for the first time in 30 years. That was a turning point.

From then on, I began weaving those fundamental movement patterns into all my therapy sessions, whether I was helping patients with joint replacements relearn left-right coordination or assisting paraplegic clients in strengthening their core for independent transfers. It was the beginning of something much bigger than I had imagined, and I felt empowered with a whole new way of approaching the treatment of Parkinson's Disease.

Word started to spread.

Kristen Gray, who ran the Jacksonville **Rock Steady Boxing** group, heard me talking about the course and invited me to teach a 16-week PWR! Moves class, *completely virtually*, to a group of people who had never had any exposure to Parkinson's Wellness Recovery exercises before. There were a lot of skeptical looks when they heard what we were going to do: "Get up from the floor without help? Exercise on my belly? Impossible!" But they did it, with the same grit and determination that I would see over and over again with people with Parkinson's.

Were they fearful? Of course. But did they let their fear stop them? No, they didn't. And because of their perseverance, at the end of 16 weeks, this group saw that they could breathe better, get up from the toilet more easily, and no longer had any fear of falling because they knew if they fell, they could get up again. All because they were willing to be brave.

This chapter is about choosing action and not letting a disease define you. It's for the person newly diagnosed and unsure of what comes next. It's for the caregiver looking for clarity. It's for the clinician or financial advisor who wants to support their client better. And above all, it's for anyone ready to turn a diagnosis into a blueprint for living with intention.

Understanding Parkinson's Disease

Parkinson's Disease (PD) is a progressive neurodegenerative disease primarily impacting movement. But to view it only through a motor lens is to miss the full picture. Parkinson's affects the whole person—physically, emotionally, cognitively, and socially.

When people first encounter a Parkinson's diagnosis, they may assume it's all about tremors or shuffling. That's the stereotype. In reality, Parkinson's Disease is nuanced and personal. In the Parkinson's community, we often say: "When you've seen one person with Parkinson's, you've seen one person with Parkinson's."

Motor Symptoms
- Bradykinesia (slowness of movement)
- Tremors (usually at rest)
- Rigidity (muscle stiffness)
- Postural instability (poor balance)
- Freezing episodes (feet "glued" to the floor)

Non-Motor Symptoms (Invisible Disabilities)
- Depression and anxiety (caused by neurochemical changes, not just sadness)
- Fatigue (even when you haven't done anything physical)
- Constipation

- Orthostatic hypotension (drop in blood pressure when standing)
- Sleep disturbances (acting out dreams due to REM disorder)
- Loss of smell
- Cognitive changes (executive function, attention)

These non-motor symptoms are just as debilitating, and quite often more distressing, than the visible ones. And yet, they're often overlooked or dismissed.

Medication vs. Movement: Why Exercise is Medicine

Most people with Parkinson's Disease are prescribed Sinemet (Carbidopa-Levodopa) to manage symptoms. It helps replace dopamine in the brain, easing movement. But it's not a cure. It's like taking Tylenol for the flu—it can help with symptoms, but it doesn't change the course of the disease.

Exercise, on the other hand, is the only intervention proven to slow progression. This is not theoretical. It's documented science. Regular physical activity triggers neuroplasticity (the brain's ability to adapt and rewire itself). It enhances mood, supports balance, improves cognition, and reduces fall risk. The Parkinson's Foundation recommends a minimum of 2.5 hours per week of moderate to intense exercise. This is not optional. It's essential.

Beyond General Exercise: Why Parkinson's-Specific Movement Matters

Exercise is essential for everyone, but for people with Parkinson's, the type of movement matters just as much as the consistency. While general activities like walking, yoga, or swimming build stamina and general health, they don't always address the specific motor and non-motor challenges of Parkinson's Disease. That's where Parkinson's-specific movement programs come in.

These programs are rooted in the brain's ability to build new pathways and change itself through practice and repetition. By focusing on amplitude, rhythm, coordination, and functional carryover, they target the very systems that Parkinson's tries to disrupt.

PWR! Moves (Parkinson's Wellness Recovery)

Developed by Dr. Becky Farley, the same neuroscientist behind LSVT BIG, PWR! Moves breaks complex movement patterns into four essential building blocks that translate directly to everyday function. These movements can be made easier or harder by doing them in sitting, standing, quadruped (on all-fours), supine (on the back), and prone (on the belly).

These four foundational movements are found in everyday actions like getting out of bed in the morning, turning your body to respond to a question, or even reacting quickly to prevent a fall. By practicing them in controlled ways, individuals build the strength, timing, and awareness they need to feel capable and confident in real life.

- **Posture & Extension**: Practicing upright movements improves balance and helps you recover from stumbles or maintain stability while walking.
- **Weight Shifting & Reaching**: Shifting side to side supports actions like buckling a seatbelt, unloading groceries, or reaching overhead.
- **Rotation & Flexibility**: Twisting through the trunk helps with rolling in bed, turning safely while walking, or putting on a jacket.

C12 | Aging in Place with Parkinson's Disease

- **Stepping & Direction Changes**: Intentional stepping supports getting in and out of cars, overcoming freezing, and safely navigating tight spaces.

These patterns translate directly into everyday tasks from dressing and driving to fall prevention. To learn more, visit www.pwr4life.org.

Urban Poling: Walking With Purpose

Urban Poling, also known as Nordic walking or pole walking, introduces an intentional, full-body rhythm to walking for people with Parkinson's. There are some incredible videos on the Urban Poling YouTube channel that show side-by-side comparisons of how much straighter and more naturally people walk, with improved arm swing, whether they're living with Parkinson's, recovering from a stroke, or healing after knee or back surgery.

The difference in function is significant, and one of the best parts is that many Urban Poling communities organize group walks, creating both physical and social benefits. I've seen how it can transform lives and that's why I became an Urban Poling Master Trainer — I wanted to be a part of training more instructors to give people a place to have fun and take care of their bodies. Why I love Urban Poling:

- ✓ **Promotes upright posture**: With something to resist against, users naturally stand taller, improving spinal alignment and reducing the common forward-stooped posture. Urban poles have the same non-slip, wide rubber tip just like a cane. Traditional hiking poles have metal tips which are great on a trail but much like walking on high heels on a sidewalk.

- ✓ **Builds core and upper body strength**: Urban Poling transforms a basic walk into a full-body workout, engaging the shoulders,

back, and core while offloading strain on knees and hips. It allows people to be able to walk longer distances by decreasing fatigue.
- ✓ **Improves balance and rhythm**: The poles offer bilateral support while encouraging rhythmic, fluid walking. This rhythm can override freezing episodes, especially when combined with the NexStride device that provides visual and auditory cues.
- ✓ **Improves confidence and mobility**: Nordic walking poles are seen in an active and positive light compared to walkers and canes. This increases usage and decreases stigma as the reason an assistive device is left behind.

Urban Poling ACTIVATOR® Poles have a patented ergonomic grip designed by an occupational therapist, eliminating the need for a tight grasp or wrist strap.

Widely used in rehabilitation, these poles support key transitional movements such as sit-to-stand and weight shifting. Lightweight, portable, and affordable, ACTIVATOR® Poles make targeted exercise accessible, no gym required. You can learn more at www.urbanpoling.com.

Environmental Strategies for Parkinson's Safety and Independence

The main goal for me when setting up the environment is to decrease the risk of falls, decrease the need for caregiver intervention, and increase independence for the person.

These are the most common interventions I recommend:

C12 | Aging in Place with Parkinson's Disease

1. Grab Bars for Stability and Cueing

- **Toilet-paper grab bar**: Provides a reminder to shift weight forward to be able to stand up and provides a secure rail to pull from if no toilet arms are available to push from.
- **Vertical bars in doorways**: Offer stability, tactile, and visual cues for automatic weight shifting in transitional areas where freezing is common. One patient described it to me as "swinging" into the bathroom. Declutter around the doorway as much as possible.
- **High color contrast reassurance rails**: Guides the person safely into the shower, with horizontal grab bars installed on all walls to provide support and stability whenever needed. For visual contrast, black or navy bars on white tile work well.
- **Ponte Giulio Vinyl-coated bars**: Offers additional grip and are warm to the touch compared to metal. Cold bars can startle patients with cognitive deficits who are often jumpy in the shower or cause pain to clients with neuropathy.

Pro Tip: For clients with cognitive challenges or slower reaction times, I recommend installing fire engine red grab bars to tap into the subconscious association of red with urgency or emergency.

- **Towel-bar grab bars**: Combine function and safety while reaching for a towel, users can steady themselves with their other hand, ensuring they're never without support.

2. Visual and Spatial Cueing

- **Bright duct tape**: Use bright duct tape or contrasting finishes to define edges of steps, table corners, or floor transitions, especially helpful for depth perception issues.

Age in Place or Find a New Space

- **Contrasting corner walls**: Painting the two walls of a corner in different colors helps trigger turning the head and body together, reducing falls from "pivot turns."
- **"Train track" targets**: Visual cues can help reduce freezing gait by giving the brain a target. Melanie told me how she laid strips of cardboard on the clinic floor to guide steps. I decided to try painter's tape for the home environment, and it worked like magic. The moment I said, *"Stomp on the blue line,"* the freezing stopped.
- **You can see it in action on my YouTube channel** *Age in Place or Find a New Space*. The video is called "How Visual and Auditory cues can decrease freezing in Parkinson's".
- **High contrast grout between tiles**: Install flooring with bigger than average spacers to create "stomp lines". You can also soften edges by using progressive shades of tiles leading up to the step line.
- **Round or square tile targets**: Plan these into the tile layout during the design phase. First, use painter's tape to test and find your ideal step distance over a few weeks, then select tile sizes to match. **Caution:** Avoid overly busy patterns, as they can trigger the vestibular system and cause dizziness!!

3. Lighting to Prevent Nighttime Falls

- **Magnetic door stops**: Keeps doors open to reduce falls and increase light on the path of travel.
- **Reassurance rails with light**: Consider **Promenaid bars** which offer an option for integrated light in their handholds.
- **Motion-activated lighting**: Install toe-kick lighting or **SnapPower** outlet nightlights to gently illuminate paths from bed to bathroom without waking others.

C12 | Aging in Place with Parkinson's Disease

- **Toilet bowl light**: Clip a motion-activated light onto the toilet rim to softly illuminate the bowl at night, improving visibility and reducing fall risk.
- **Under-bed motion sensor**–Place a driveway alarm sensor under the bed so it chimes when feet hit the floor. Especially useful when caregivers sleep in a different room or during post-anesthesia confusion (e.g., after colonoscopies).
  - *Pro tip:* If needed, you can muffle the speaker with a sock to reduce the volume for nighttime use.

4. Bedside Safety and Transfers

- **Half bed rails**: Prevent falls out of bed and provide a sturdy handhold for getting in and out using cues like "nose over toes" and "bottom in the air."
- **Injury prevention flooring**: To minimize injury with REM disorder, you can buy beveled fall mats like Smart Cells, gym floor mats, or thick yoga mats. The important thing is to ensure that the edges are taped down with color-contrast tape to prevent tripping on them.
- **Raizer**: A portable, battery-operated lifting chair that helps safely raise a person from the floor to a seated position with minimal physical effort from the caregiver.
- **Raymex**: A compact, floor-to-standing walker that provides sturdy handgrips and step supports to help individuals safely get up from the floor with minimal assistance.

5. Smart Alerts and Motion Sensors

- **Discreet alerts for privacy and safety:** Smart sensors can notify caregivers when the person is on the move, without hovering or interrupting.
- **For a low-tech option**: use wireless doorbells with plug-in transmitters around the home or yard to signal movement.

6. Mirrors for Visual Feedback

- A common challenge for people with Parkinson's is the overestimation of their movements. They may feel like they're lifting their leg high enough to clear sidewalk curbs or shower thresholds, but in reality, they may only be lifting it a few inches.
- In this case, sometimes the fall is due to stiffness in the neck or slow eye muscles, making it hard to look down to see where to step off the curb. Some people will say "Curb!" out loud to activate muscles and remind themselves to look down.
- One practical solution is to incorporate mirrors throughout the home, allowing individuals to visually monitor and adjust their posture and movements in real time. This helps retrain the brain to better understand where their limbs actually are in space compared to where they *feel* they are, a critical aspect of proprioception.

7. Anti-Constipation

- Slowness of movements includes the bowels. The ideal biomechanics of a bowel movement is to have the knees as high as possible compared to the hips. This can be difficult if a person has arthritic knees or weakness in the quads that make it harder to go from sitting to standing.
- Adding a **Squatty Potty** can help get into the right position, and adding toilet arms can help to push up from the toilet seat.
- Some clients find that the spray of a bidet can help to stimulate bowel movements. Generally, I find that routines are the most helpful to teach the body what to do. Wake up, eat, drink, exercise, and then 20 to 40 minutes later, plan to spend some time in the bathroom.

C12 | Aging in Place with Parkinson's Disease

Parkinson's-Specific Product Ideas

"Stop stealing their therapy!" This is my favorite reminder to well-meaning caregivers who express love by doing everything for the person they care about. But here's the thing—every button they fasten, every step they help with, every spoon they lift is an opportunity taken from the person to practice and maintain their independence.

Instead of removing those challenges, let's support them with tools that enable independence. The right products can reduce frustration, promote dignity, and even improve safety, but I know trying to find the ones that are best for you can be overwhelming. A single Google search might yield thousands of results with no clear direction.

To help you get started, I've put together a list of common challenges and some example products. Use these as a springboard so you can begin your own search with confidence, armed with the right keywords and use-cases. Whether you're a caregiver, professional, or someone navigating Parkinson's yourself, the right solution may be just one idea away.

1. Gait and Movement Support

- **What it solves**: Freezing, shuffling, and difficulty initiating movement.
- **Try searching for**: "Laser shoes for Parkinson's", "Visual cue walker."
- **Example products**:
    - **NexStride**: a portable device that attaches to a cane or walker to provide laser and metronome cues that help break freezing episodes.
    - **U-Step Walker**: A mobility device with reverse brakes for safety and built-in laser and metronome cues to help break freezing episodes and improve walking rhythm.
    - **Walk with Path**: Laser cueing shoes with a visual line for freezing episodes and to improve step initiation.

2. Bed Mobility

- **What it solves**: Difficulty repositioning in bed due to stiffness or tangled sheets
- **Try searching for**: "Friction-reducing sheets," "Zip-in bedding."
- **Example products**:
    - **Comfort Linen**: Ultra-smooth sheet and pajama system that reduces friction and allows users to reposition independently. Edges are grippy to prevent slipping off the bed. 80% of their sales are to people with Parkinson's!!
    - **Beddy's**: Zippered all-in-one bedding that makes it easy to get in and out of bed and keeps covers in place, ideal for those with limited mobility or dexterity.

3. Tremor Management and Eating

- **What it solves**: Dropping utensils, spilling food, loss of appetite.
- **Try searching for**: "Weighted utensils for Parkinson's," "Adaptive plates for tremors."
- **Example products**:
    - **Steadiwear**: A lightweight, battery-free glove designed to stabilize hand tremors in real time, helping users perform daily tasks like eating and drinking.
    - **Obi Robots**: A robotic feeding device that allows users to eat independently by controlling the robotic arm with simple switches.
    - **Pasta-style bowls with high sides or plate guards**: Keep food on the utensil longer; some attractive versions are now available on Amazon.

C12 | Aging in Place with Parkinson's Disease

4. Fine Motor Dressing Aids

- **What it solves**: Trouble with buttons, zippers, or bras.
- **Try searching for**: "Adaptive clothing Parkinson's," "One-handed dressing tools."
- **Example products**:
    - **Springrose Bras**–Beautiful, easy-to-fasten bras designed for women with limited dexterity.
    - **Joe & Bella**–Stylish, adaptive clothing designed for comfort, dignity, and ease of dressing for older adults and caregivers.
    - **MagnaReady**–Button-up shirts with magnetic closures that look like traditional buttons, making dressing easier for people with limited mobility or dexterity.

5. Health Tracking and Monitoring

- **What it solves**: Medication timing, monitoring motor fluctuations.
- **Try searching for**: "Parkinson's tracking app," "Smartwatch for PD."
- **Example products**:
    - **NeuroRPM**–An FDA-cleared app that uses Apple Watch sensors to passively monitor tremors, gait, mobility patterns, and symptom severity, providing real-time data to clinicians to guide personalized treatment.
    - **StrivePD**–An app that uses Apple Watch to track tremors, medication schedules, and symptom trends to help patients and clinicians personalize care based on real-time data.

6. Environmental Control and Safety

- **What it solves**: Fall risk, late-night disorientation, appliance safety
- **Try searching for**: "Motion sensor lighting," "Smart stove knob."
- **Example ideas**:
  - **Voice-activated lights** (e.g., Alexa + smart bulbs). *Note: You can enable Whisper Mode on Alexa, which allows her to listen and respond at a lower, quieter volume.*
  - **Stove shutoff devices** with timer-based controls like **Ome Kitchen**, or movement-based, like **iGuard**.
  - **No WiFi options to control lights** like **Lotus Ring**.

7. Functional Seating and Transfers

- **What it solves**: Additional support during transitions
- **Try searching for**: "Lift chair," "Comfort height toilet," "Toilet paper grab bars."
- **Example ideas**:
  - **Golden lift chairs** for adjustable sleeping and recline support.
  - **Bemis Assurance** for raised toilet seat, armrests, and bidet.
  - **Toilet paper holders with built-in grab bars** to assist during descent.

Moving Water Can't Freeze

I want to end this chapter by emphasizing how vital exercise is to the quality of life for someone with Parkinson's disease. Exercise doesn't just slow the progression. It actively helps break up abnormal movement patterns, allowing you to function better in everyday life. And just like a waterfall, if you stay in motion, you'll never freeze.

C12 | Aging in Place with Parkinson's Disease

Morning Stretches

Simple stretches that counteract the stiff extension common in Parkinson's can be done right in bed and can make a big difference in a person's ability to bend forward to stand up from the edge of the bed.

The goal is to promote flexion to balance the overnight stiffness and extension that Parkinson's often causes. Anything that encourages the motions needed to curl into a ball is a win. I recommend building these stretches into a morning routine so they become automatic, just part of how you start the day.

Here's an example of a sequence many patients find easy to integrate:

- Bring one knee toward the chest, hold the stretch for 20 seconds, then repeat on the other side.
- Bring both knees toward the chest and tuck the chin to form a ball, holding the position for 20 seconds.
- Lie on the bed with arms outstretched and knees bent together. Gently let your knees fall to one side while turning your head to the opposite side. Repeat on the other side.
- Now lie like a starfish, with both arms and legs spread out as far as possible. Turn your head to the right to look at your right hand. Then stretch your entire body to the right, as if you're reaching for an apple just out of reach. Really try to engage your whole body in the stretch.
- While sitting on the edge of the bed, ideally next to a bedrail, run your hands down your legs until you feel a good stretch. When you reach that point, extend your hands forward as if you're trying to touch the wall, focusing on stretching each vertebra in your spine—imagine you're on a medieval stretching machine. Hold the stretch for a few seconds, then quickly pull yourself back up to sitting, making sure to engage your back and stomach muscles. Repeat five times.
- Scoot your bottom to the edge of the bed, making sure your feet are firmly planted on the floor, shoulder width apart and ready to

bear weight. With your arms on the bed, lean your weight forward into "Nose over Toes" position and push yourself up to standing in one quick motion to teach your muscles to react faster. Repeat five times.

Find Your Tribe

Non-motor symptoms like fatigue, pain, depression, and apathy are part of the neurochemical changes that occur in Parkinson's, and many report that battling these is the hardest obstacle to overcome. The key to not letting these symptoms take over is finding a community to exercise with because staying active is easier and more enjoyable when you don't do it alone.

Why is this such a vital part of the Parkinson's journey? Research shows that the level of exertion needed to slow the progression of the disease is where it's not comfortable to talk and exercise. Consistently maintaining that high level of intensity is not an easy thing to motivate yourself to do, day in and day out.

But when your exercise class is really about meeting up with your friends at a Rock Steady Boxing group three times a week, it simply becomes the activity you do together. The best part? Your tribe will be the ones calling you when you don't show up. The Parkinson's community is incredibly active, with many Parkinson's-specific exercise groups available, including yoga, tai chi, dancing, cycling, and even singing.

Final Thoughts

Parkinson's may change the roadmap, but it doesn't erase the journey. Throughout this chapter, we've explored how understanding the disease, its visible symptoms, hidden challenges, and evolving treatments can shift the narrative from fear to possibility.

Whether you are newly diagnosed, caring for someone you love, or supporting clients as a professional, remember this: knowledge is

C12 | Aging in Place with Parkinson's Disease

power, and movement is medicine. Every day, new solutions are emerging from wearable tech to targeted exercise programs to smart home modifications.

Don't let overwhelm stop you from trying new things. You don't have to do everything at once. You just have to start. Choose one thing to try. Ask one new question. Take one bold step forward.

The truth is this isn't about fighting Parkinson's. It's about living with it, on your terms. When you have the right tools, the right mindset, and a supportive team behind you, you can age in place with strength, dignity, and hope. Keep learning. Keep adapting. Keep going. You've got this.

A Tribute to Bill Wilson

"Parkinson's is a relentless fighter who never slows down. It is hard to keep from allowing it to guide your life. But it can be done. Resist the temptation to stay in bed. Resist the temptation to avoid exercise class because it's raining. Resist all the other things that Parkinson's throws at you."

--Bill Wilson

Bill Wilson was an extraordinary advocate and friend to the Jacksonville Parkinson's community. His tireless leadership, generosity, and ability to bring people together created a space where individuals with Parkinson's and their families felt truly seen, supported, and empowered. Bill didn't just build connections—he built a community rooted in hope, compassion, and resilience. I dedicate this chapter to Bill—a patient, a friend, and someone who taught me so much about Parkinson's disease and what it means to live with purpose and grace.

Box 3

Age in Place or Find a New Space

Key Takeaways

- Parkinson's is now the second-fastest-growing neurological condition in the world.
- Empathy begins with understanding both motor and non-motor symptoms.
- Medication manages symptoms, but only exercise slows progression.
- PWR! Moves and Urban Poling target the unique challenges of Parkinson's.
- Small environmental tweaks can reduce fall risk and caregiver strain.
- Innovative tools restore confidence and support daily function.
- Stay curious—new solutions are emerging every day.

Chapter Thirteen

Epilogue

Years ago, when I was mentoring a young occupational therapist on all the ways she could provide exceptional care to patients in the home environment, she turned to me mid-scribble in her now over-filled notebook and said to me in an exasperated voice, "This is completely impossible. I'm just going to have to figure out how to download everything from your brain into my brain." Technological advances are being explored on how individuals can control a computer with only their thoughts, so perhaps one day, this will indeed be possible.

Until then, my hope is that this book offers you a glimpse into how I think and how I see the world a little differently. Maybe it's my love of solving problems or my drive to tackle a challenge, but throughout my life, I've always found myself raising my hand to take on the cases that others had given up on.

For many years, I ran a highly specialized private practice focused on persistent pain cases—patients who had spent years pursuing every possible treatment with all types of specialists.

Age in Place or Find a New Space

Most of these patients were middle-aged, active, and otherwise healthy individuals who had followed the standard course of care. They were referred to me because, despite regaining about 75 percent of their function, it was that remaining 25 percent that held them back from returning to the activities they truly loved—the things that made their lives meaningful.

I approached those cases in the same way you've seen throughout this book, with a blank slate. I start by asking a million questions, sometimes for forty-five uninterrupted minutes before I even begin to examine the site of injury.

I ask about the quality of their pain, the activities that aggravate it, and what, if anything, makes it better. I ask how their pain affects their ability to dress, bathe, groom, cook, clean, do laundry, and perform their jobs. I ask about their typical day, their stress levels, how they unwind, what they enjoy for fun, and how they stay connected with family and friends.

All of these questions help me build a complete picture of the person sitting in front of me and offer valuable insight into what truly matters to them and what will genuinely motivate them to do the work to get better.

When I begin, I don't pretend to have all the answers. I am always upfront with my patients. I don't have a magic wand or a crystal ball to predict the future. I would never claim with certainty that a specific exercise or treatment protocol is the definitive solution.

What I do know is that through asking big-picture, thirty-thousand-foot-view questions, I begin to see patterns—patterns of pain, of asymmetry, of what might be driving the problem beneath the surface.

I share what I observe and offer my perspective on potential treatment options. I give my honest opinion about which path I believe holds the greatest potential impact. I discuss the pros and cons, including the potential costs to the client in time, money, and effort.

I lay out a roadmap with possible directions and let them choose the first step that best aligns with their personality and preferences.

C13 | Epilogue

Sometimes that sounds like, "There's no way I can fit that into my day all at once, but maybe I can break it up and do some of it on my drive to the office." We take one step, then reassess and decide if we want to continue in that direction. Then we take another step. And repeat.

This strategy has proven successful for me as I problem-solve through both why pain continues to affect a person's life and why people resist changes that seem like no-brainers. I hope this approach will work for you too.

I have been inspired by many wonderful patients who have touched and changed my life through my interactions with them. Writing this book is my way of paying that kindness forward, offering ideas to help ease the stress and overwhelm I see unfolding in families across the world.

Older adults and their families need support, not just from their inner circles, but also from their communities and governments at large. My work as an occupational therapist in the home setting has given me a front-row seat to witness the suffering and hard consequences that come from not saving enough, not prioritizing health and exercise, and not preparing adequately for the natural changes that come with aging.

My hope is that we can do better to stop this cycle and to create a more supportive future for all of us.

The Four Cornerstones of Thriving at Home

Throughout this book, we've explored the four essential cornerstones of aging in place: home modification, physical fitness, lifestyle medicine, and technology. These cornerstones are not isolated. They are interconnected, forming the foundation of a life where you can truly thrive at home.

- **Home modification** is more than grab bars and ramps, it's about crafting spaces that support your routines, your passions, and your

connections. Every thoughtful design choice is an investment in your future independence.
- **Physical fitness** is the currency of aging. It keeps you strong, mobile, and able to participate in the moments that matter most. Movement is not just a medical prescription. It's the key to protecting the life you love.
- **Lifestyle medicine** reminds us that our habits today shape our health tomorrow. The foods we choose, the routines we keep, the quality of our sleep, and the strength of our social ties all play powerful roles in determining how we age.
- **Technology** is our silent partner. From smart homes that prevent falls to devices that connect us to loved ones across distances, technology can help us age safely, stay engaged, and make our homes work for us, not against us.

When nurtured together, these cornerstones create a life where aging in place is not only possible—it's vibrant, joyful, and sustainable.

Preparing, Not Just Planning

One of the most important lessons in this book is that planning is not enough. Preparation is key. Planning is deciding where you want to go. Preparation involves packing your bags, mapping your route, and having a contingency plan for rainy days.

Aging in place starts earlier than most people think. Every remodel is an opportunity to build universal design features. Every healthy habit you start now becomes a gift to your future self. By preparing early, you give yourself and your loved ones the freedom to navigate aging with confidence, not crisis.

C13 | Epilogue

Caregiving: The Heart of Aging in Place

We cannot talk about aging without honoring caregivers. Whether you are a caregiver, have been one, or will one day rely on one, this journey touches us all. Caregiving is not just about tasks. It's about relationships, dignity, and shared humanity.

You don't have to do this alone. There are resources, teams, and support systems that can help carry the weight. Organizations like AARP Caregiving offer practical tools and connection points to guide you through the process. The beauty of caregiving today is that you have options: technology can offer peace of mind, communities can offer social support, and thoughtful preparation can give everyone room to breathe.

The Global Aging Shift: An Invitation to Innovate

Around the world, populations are aging faster than systems can keep up. Japan has already crossed the threshold with nearly 30 percent of its population over age 65. The global aging crisis is here, and healthcare systems, housing markets, and family structures are being tested in ways we've never seen before.

What will it look like when people are living longer, but with fewer caregivers available? Can technology bridge the gap? Can design get ahead of the need? If we're going to meet the challenge of global aging, we must think much bigger.

At events like Consumer Electronics Show (CES), I've seen AgeTech changing the game with wearable fall detection, home sensors that track daily activity, voice-activated health monitoring, smart toilets, assistive robots, and virtual rehabilitation.

But innovation isn't just about high-tech, it starts in everyday life. Countries, companies, startups, and caregivers must work together to identify the problems at the root, share the knowledge of what's working, and stop duplicating efforts that go nowhere. We don't need a hundred tools that do the same thing. We need smart, beautiful, validated solutions that work—and fast. Caregivers needed help yesterday.

Healthy Habits Are Free

While technology can help us scale, the most important thing to recognize is that the most impactful interventions are free: sleep, hydration, movement, breath, and mindset. You can't age in place if you're in and out of the hospital with unmanaged conditions. Grab bars can't fix chronic dehydration. Fall alarms can't fix missed medications. The foundation is lifestyle medicine. This is where participation matters most. The secret to aging well is showing up for yourself today.

Final Thoughts: Your Next Step Starts Today

Thank you for taking this journey with me. I hope you feel empowered, prepared, and inspired to build a life full of meaningful conversations, laughter around the kitchen table, and experience lots of hugs from grandchildren. The home you design, the habits you build, and the conversations you have will ripple through your life and through the lives of those who love you.

You can shape your future with intention, creativity, and joy. Your environment can be your partner in living well, not just a place where you grow old. And when we approach conversations around aging with open hearts and compassion, we all win.

So, what's next?

Start where you are. Start today. Your next step might be as small as adding a suction grab bar or starting a walking routine. Maybe it's making that financial planning appointment or having the hard conversation with your family about what really matters to you.

You can do this—I believe in you. We'll walk this journey together, one step at a time.

One Last Thing...

How I Practice What I Preach: Staying Ready for the Next Adventure

Staying healthy and strong isn't just something I talk about - it's a driving force in my life. For me, movement and exploration go hand in hand.

I love to travel and I love to learn. I've backpacked through remote trails in the hills of Vietnam, hiked gorges in China, climbed Mount Kilimanjaro in Africa, danced during Carnaval in Brazil, trained with national teams in the South of France, visited fortresses in Spain, and scuba-dived in the crystal-clear waters of the Philippines, Indonesia and Thailand. These aren't just travel stories. They're the result of years of being intentional and open to whatever is next.

The person who most shaped how I think about aging and adventure was someone I met while backpacking in my twenties. Back then, I was taking local buses, sleeping in hostels, hopping in and out of boats to reach islands before all the rooms were gone, sometimes facing the possibility of sleeping on the beach if I didn't move quickly enough. It was a time of pure adventure.

Age in Place or Find a New Space

That's when I noticed him - a man in his mid-sixties traveling solo alongside twenty-somethings. It was unusual to see someone his age taking local transport, figuring things out on the fly, and moving between boats, buses, and backroads like the rest of us. One day, I finally sat down and had a long conversation with him. I asked what it was like to travel in your sixties because deep down, I wanted that life for myself too.

He told me his secret: every year before his annual two-month backpacking trip, he would remove one piece of clothing from his pack for every year he aged. When I met him at sixty-six, he was down to just two shirts: the one on his back and one in his pack. He chose quick-dry, lightweight clothing so he could wash them each night and always be ready to move. His story wasn't about packing light. It was about intentionally evaluating what really matters each year.

What stuck with me most was how much this style of travel kept him sharp. He wasn't sitting comfortably on a tour bus waiting to be told where to shop or where to eat. He was figuring out which bus to catch in a foreign language, how much it cost, and where it was going. He was making backup plans, watching for pickpockets, thinking several steps ahead. Travel wasn't just physical for him, it was a daily mental exercise in flexibility and problem-solving.

That way of thinking shaped how I approached not only travel but life. I learned that everything is manageable when you break it into steps. Climbing Kilimanjaro can seem overwhelming if you look at the summit on day one. But when you take it one section at a time—today is the rainforest, tomorrow the rocky slope—it's just about taking the next step. Sometimes all you need to do is keep your eyes on the trail directly in front of you, looking up every now and then to make sure you're still heading in the right direction.

I also met people along the way who deepened this lesson. An older couple told me, "Even if you end up just working as a Walmart greeter later in life, you'll still have these memories in your head, memories no one can take away." I met parents carrying children along

One Last Thing . . . How I Practice What I Preach

steep mountain trails, showing me that with enough planning, persistence, and willingness to figure it out step by step, most things are possible.

Even when I look back at those days—traveling without smartphones, tracking local embassies in case my passport was stolen, sending emails from internet cafés that took 40 minutes to load—I see now that those experiences gave me tools I still use. They taught me the importance of staying active, staying mentally engaged, and always having something to look forward to.

This is why I practice what I preach. Staying healthy isn't just about living longer. It's about staying ready for the next adventure, whatever that might be. It's about moving through life with curiosity, adaptability, and purpose. That's what fuels me, and that's what I hope to pass along.

You can find interviews, resources and downloads for the following PDFs on my website at **www.EvolvingHomes.com**.

Please feel free to share them with anyone that could benefit. When we work together, we all win ☺

****

Author's Note:

This book was written as a passion project in hopes that equitable access to knowledge could lead to healthier people, happier families and vibrant communities.

If you enjoyed this book, please consider leaving a review so that others may benefit from these resources too. Thank you ☺

Appendix A: Tools & Resources

Hospital to Home Checklist

Car to Wheelchair / Walker
- Are they able to pivot and get legs out?
- Do I need to prevent sliding off the seat?
- Can they go sit to stand from the seat?
- Is there a way to get them in if it's raining?

Through the Front Door
- is there a clear path to get to the house?
- does the wheelchair fit through the door?
- Do I need a ramp or threshold?

Into the Bathroom
- Is the door wide enough to get through?
- Can the door come off the hinges?
- Is there space to put in offset hinges?
- Do they need a grab bar for the transfer?
- Is there space to help transfer to toilet?
- Is the height of the toilet level with WC?
- Will they be able to clean themselves?
- can they alert me if they need help?
- Does the light come on automatically?

Into the Shower
- Do they need a grab bar to get in/ out?
- Is there a place to sit to bathe?
- Can they reach the shampoo/ Soap safely?
- Is there a shower hose with pause button?
- Where will they put the shower hose when not in use?

Into the Bed
- Is there space next to the bed to transfer?
- Is there a rail to hold onto to get in?
- Can they get in/out safely?
- Can they sit on edge of the bed securely?
- Is the path to the bathroom clear?
- Can they alert you if they need help?

EvolvingHomes.com
We help caregivers navigate difficult decisions confidently.

Appendix A | Tools & Resources

30 day water challenge

#		#	
1	🥛🥛🥛🥛🥛🥛🥛🥛	16	🥛🥛🥛🥛🥛🥛🥛🥛
2	🥛🥛🥛🥛🥛🥛🥛🥛	17	🥛🥛🥛🥛🥛🥛🥛🥛
3	🥛🥛🥛🥛🥛🥛🥛🥛	18	🥛🥛🥛🥛🥛🥛🥛🥛
4	🥛🥛🥛🥛🥛🥛🥛🥛	19	🥛🥛🥛🥛🥛🥛🥛🥛
5	🥛🥛🥛🥛🥛🥛🥛🥛	20	🥛🥛🥛🥛🥛🥛🥛🥛
6	🥛🥛🥛🥛🥛🥛🥛🥛	21	🥛🥛🥛🥛🥛🥛🥛🥛
7	🥛🥛🥛🥛🥛🥛🥛🥛	22	🥛🥛🥛🥛🥛🥛🥛🥛
8	🥛🥛🥛🥛🥛🥛🥛🥛	23	🥛🥛🥛🥛🥛🥛🥛🥛
9	🥛🥛🥛🥛🥛🥛🥛🥛	24	🥛🥛🥛🥛🥛🥛🥛🥛
10	🥛🥛🥛🥛🥛🥛🥛🥛	25	🥛🥛🥛🥛🥛🥛🥛🥛
11	🥛🥛🥛🥛🥛🥛🥛🥛	26	🥛🥛🥛🥛🥛🥛🥛🥛
12	🥛🥛🥛🥛🥛🥛🥛🥛	27	🥛🥛🥛🥛🥛🥛🥛🥛
13	🥛🥛🥛🥛🥛🥛🥛🥛	28	🥛🥛🥛🥛🥛🥛🥛🥛
14	🥛🥛🥛🥛🥛🥛🥛🥛	29	🥛🥛🥛🥛🥛🥛🥛🥛
15	🥛🥛🥛🥛🥛🥛🥛🥛	30	🥛🥛🥛🥛🥛🥛🥛🥛

The Secrets to Healthy Aging are all FREE!!
Water, Sleep, Exercise!

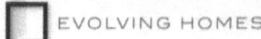 EVOLVING HOMES

We help homeowners create Aging-in-Place Plans!
EvolvingHomes.com

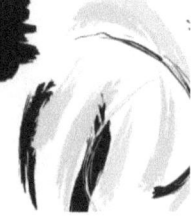

Age in Place or Find a New Space

BUILDING HEALTHY HABITS:
30 DAY MOVEMENT CHALLENGE

1 WALK	2 Try something new!	3 WALK	4 Family Activity	5 WALK
6 WALK	7 Try something new!	8 WALK	9 Family Activity	10 WALK
11 WALK	12 Try something new!	13 WALK	14 Family Activity	15 WALK
16 WALK	17 Try something new!	18 WALK	19 Family Activity	20 WALK
21 WALK	22 Try something new!	23 WALK	24 Family Activity	25 WALK
26 WALK	27 Try something new!	28 WALK	29 Family Activity	30 WALK

MY WHY: (WRITE YOUR GOAL!)

Appendix A | Tools & Resources

EVOLVING HOMES

30 DAY CHALLENGE VITALS LOG

MONTH: YEAR:

DATE	TIME	PRESSURE	PULSE	OXYGEN

EvolvingHomes.com

Age in Place or Find a New Space

MY DAILY ROUTINE

ROUTINES ARE IMPORTANT TO FEEL YOUR BEST!

EVOLVING HOMES

PICK A CONSISTENT WAKE-UP TIME (EVEN IF YOU NAP LATER) TO START THE CLOCK SO YOUR BODY KNOWS WHEN TO EXPECT MEDS + FOOD.

SCHEDULE	MORNING ROUTINE
6 AM	•
7 AM	•
8 AM	•
9 AM	•
10 AM	•
11 AM	•
12 PM	**EVENING ROUTINE**
1 PM	
2 PM	
3 PM	
4 PM	
5 PM	
6 PM	**EXERCISES**
7 PM	
8 PM	
9 PM	

Appendix A | Tools & Resources

Myofascial Stress & Pain Relief

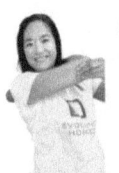

(1) Upper Back & Shoulder

Find a tender spot & cross your hands over your chest.

Move up and down slowly, massaging knots or tender areas.

(2) Chest & Shoulders

Face the wall. & place ball on chest close to your armpit.

Lean forward and slowly roll the ball on the chest and shoulder area.

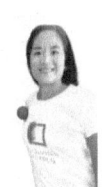

(3) Lower Back & Glutes

Place ball and roll up and down, side to side until you •find a tender spot.

Relax your weight into the wall, allowing the ball to apply pressure for 30 sec

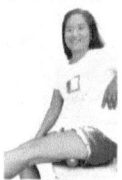

(4) Hamstring Kicks

Sit on a hard surface & place ball under leg.

Lean forward to put body weight onto leg.. Slowly kick your leg forward 5x

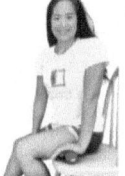

(5) Acupressure Hands & Feet

Place ball under arch of foot or palm of hand. Put weight into ball and make 30 circles. Lift toes or fingers up 5x.

Lean weight forwards and roll ball back and forth on arch.

Age in Place or Find a New Space

8 WEEK SCHEDULE

	WALKING	ACTIVE LIVING	8 CUPS WATER/DAY
Week 1	Monday: DONE! @ __:__ Thursday: DONE! @ __:__	Tuesday: DONE! @ __:__ Friday: DONE! @ __:__	M T W Th F
Week 2	Monday: DONE! @ __:__ Thursday: DONE! @ __:__	Tuesday: DONE! @ __:__ Friday: DONE! @ __:__	M T W Th F
Week 3	Monday: DONE! @ __:__ Thursday: DONE! @ __:__	Tuesday: DONE! @ __:__ Friday: DONE! @ __:__	M T W Th F
Week 4	Monday: DONE! @ __:__ Thursday: DONE! @ __:__	Tuesday: DONE! @ __:__ Friday: DONE! @ __:__	M T W Th F
Week 5	Monday: DONE! @ __:__ Thursday: DONE! @ __:__	Tuesday: DONE! @ __:__ Friday: DONE! @ __:__	M T W Th F
Week 6	Monday: DONE! @ __:__ Thursday: DONE! @ __:__	Tuesday: DONE! @ __:__ Friday: DONE! @ __:__	M T W Th F
Week 7	Monday: DONE! @ __:__ Thursday: DONE! @ __:__	Tuesday: DONE! @ __:__ Friday: DONE! @ __:__	M T W Th F
Week 8	Monday: DONE! @ __:__ Thursday: DONE! @ __:__	Tuesday: DONE! @ __:__ Friday: DONE! @ __:__	M T W Th F

EvolvingHomes.com

Appendix A | Tools & Resources

Age in Place or Find a New Space®: Planning Tool

Use this tool to compare your real options and make confident, informed decisions—on your own timeline.

Step 1: Clarify Your Non-Negotiables

Ask yourself:
- Do I want to stay in my current neighborhood or city?
- How important is proximity to family, friends, healthcare, or community?
- How much space do I need to feel comfortable?
- What activities and routines do I want to support in my next chapter?

Write your top 3 non-negotiables:
1.
2.
3.

Step 2: Evaluate Your Current Home

Use contractor quotes or a home assessment (with an OT if possible) to understand:
- What modifications are needed?
- How much will they cost?
- How disruptive will the process be?

Summary of needed modifications: _____
Estimated cost: _____
Projected timeline: _____

Age in Place or Find a New Space

Step 3: Research Local Alternatives

Visit open houses, 55+ communities, and continuing care communities in your area and in other locations you'd realistically consider (e.g. closer to family).

For each home or community, document:

- ✓ Option: _____
- ✓ Location: _____
- ✓ Pros: _____
- ✓ Cons: _____
- ✓ Size (sq. ft): _____
- ✓ Needed Modifications: _____
- ✓ Estimated Cost (Home + Reno): _____

Step 4: Compare Apples to Apples

Now compare:
- Renovating your current home
- Moving to another home in your area
- Exploring other housing models (e.g., CCRC, new build in 55+)

Use total cost (purchase + modification), not just listing prices.

Which option gives you:
- The best fit for your needs?
- The least stress during transition?
- The most long-term flexibility?

Step 5: Reflect Before You Decide

Ask yourself:
- If I choose this path, will I feel relieved or unsure?
- Am I acting from fear, pressure, or clarity and intention?
- Do I feel peace with this decision?

Appendix A | Tools & Resources

Alternative Living Options

1. Independent Living Communities (ILCs)
For older adults who are still fairly active but need a more supportive environment, free of home maintenance responsibilities.
- No medical care provided.
- Meals, housekeeping, and social activities are often included.
- Ideal for seniors who are socially isolated but don't need daily assistance.

Not regulated as healthcare facilities.
Also known as: Retirement community, senior apartment, 55+ housing

2. Assisted Living Facilities (ALFs)
For those who need help with daily tasks like bathing, dressing, medication reminders, or meals—but not full-time nursing care.
- Staff available 24/7 for personal care.
- Residents have private or semi-private apartments.
- Often includes activities, transportation, and dining services.

Regulated by each state/province (varies widely).

3. Memory Care Units (within ALFs or separate)
Designed for individuals with Alzheimer's disease or other forms of dementia who may need secure environments and specialized support.
- Trained staff and secure facilities to prevent wandering.
- Structured daily routines and sensory activities.
- Higher staff-to-resident ratio than typical ALFs.

Often, a specialized wing of an assisted living or nursing facility.

4. Skilled Nursing Facilities (SNFs) / Nursing Homes
Provide 24/7 medical care, rehabilitation, and personal assistance for those with complex or chronic health needs.
- On-site licensed nurses and therapists

Age in Place or Find a New Space

- May be long-term or short-term (after hospitalization)
- Medicare/Medicaid may help cover costs

Heavily regulated, medical model.

5. Continuing Care Retirement Communities (CCRCs)

Offer multiple levels of care in one location, so residents can transition from independent to assisted to nursing care without leaving the community.

- "Aging in place" within a single campus
- Often requires a large upfront fee
- Great for long-term planning and minimizing moves

Some nonprofit, others for-profit.

6. Adult Foster Homes / Adult Family Homes / Board & Care Homes

Small, residential settings where 4–6 residents live together and receive personal care from live-in or on-site staff.

- Homelike atmosphere, often more personalized care
- Often less expensive than ALFs or SNFs
- May not be available in every state or country

Licensing and oversight vary by region.

7. Shared Housing / Co-Housing / Home Sharing

Living with another adult or caregiver in exchange for rent, care, or companionship. Sometimes facilitated by nonprofits.

- Ideal for those who are semi-independent but need supervision or help.
- Can be informal (family/friends) or through formal programs.
- Growing trend in urban areas.

Alternative aging model gaining traction.

Appendix A | Tools & Resources

8. Hospice or Palliative Residential Homes

For end-of-life care when hospital or home care is no longer appropriate.
- Focused on comfort, dignity, and pain management
- Often includes emotional, spiritual, and family support
- May be covered by Medicare or national healthcare plans

Usually nonprofit or hospital-affiliated.

Questions to Ask After a Fall

Mom's had a fall... now what?

Hearing these words can be terrifying for adult children. When someone you love falls for the first time, the first thing people feel is often disbelief. "Oh my goodness, are they ok? What happened? They've always been so independent and in such great shape."

Sometimes people feel guilty. Was there something I could've done to prevent this? Did she fall because I haven't been spending enough time there? Maybe I've been neglecting her needs and didn't notice that she's been getting weaker.

So many questions, not enough answers.

Most often, people feel fearful and at a loss for what to do. So they do what we all do and ask Google. They need solutions, but instead, often end up with more questions than answers.

Many just feel even more overwhelmed with the search results.

Does she need grab bars? But if she needs grab bars, she will never let me do that! She is so proud of her home.

Maybe she just needs to have someone with her at all times? But this person on Facebook says it costs their family $20,000 a month! That's crazy! We can't afford that!

Maybe it's time for her to consider assisted living? But wait, I can't find out what the cost is unless I tour each and every one of them to find out what their current promotions are? I'm in California and she's in Florida. What *now*?

Cue the swirling emotions of overwhelm.

Take a Deep Breath

Let's put all that aside for just a minute. First, breathe. There's no need to panic and definitely no need to take someone else's experience and assume that will be yours.

Appendix A | Tools & Resources

There's a very big difference in the level of care needed between someone who was previously healthy and active versus somebody who has been sick for years with chronic illnesses and has NEVER exercised.

There is also a huge range of potential solutions depending on the variables. More options isn't always better. For example, Arms on the shower chair are great for someone with arthritic knees that need help from the arms to get up but can be a significant fall risk for someone who has visual issues or left neglect from a stroke that might cause them to bump into the armrest and lose their balance.

Ask the Right Questions

A better way to figure out what is needed is by formulating the right questions. The only way to get on the right track for the right solution is to understand how they got there.

Here's where to start:

Find out what happened.
- Was this just a fluke accident?
- Was that baking dish just too high, and that's why they fell backwards? Did they genuinely not notice that there was another step?
- Did the dog see a squirrel and pulled them forward?
- Did they have a fall in the shower because they were dizzy? Did they fall in the bedroom, rushing to get to the bathroom before they had an accident?
- Did they turn on the lights when they entered a room?
- The more details you can gather, the more information you'll have to understand the reason behind it and if this is an easily solvable one or not.

Are their vitals good?

Age in Place or Find a New Space

- When was the last time they had a physical done? Are there medical issues that need to be addressed that they haven't gotten around to yet?
- Have they had their vision checked? Do they notice more stumbles when they are going to the bathroom in the middle of the night?
- You're looking for what's different than their normal independent self.

How are they physically?
- Are they feeling weaker? Are they in pain? Are they needing more help Day to day?
- Have they noticed things getting harder to do, like getting in and out of bed?
- Are they still doing all the things they used to?
- Are they exercising? How are they staying strong?
- Did they used to go to the gym three days a week but can't now due to COVID-19?

Is pain stopping them from exercising?
- Did they used to walk with their friends, but their knees are hurting too much now?
- Maybe they hurt their back lifting something out of the trunk of their car, and that pain is still not resolved, so they're not back to their normal routine.
- Ask if pain is the reason someone has stopped a favorite activity. If it's not getting better on its own after a few weeks, it's definitely worth discussing with your doctor before the inactivity makes you weak enough to be at risk of more falls.

You are looking for any circumstances that have stopped them from being able to stay as active as they usually are.

Appendix A | Tools & Resources

Are they taking good care of themselves?
- What are their lifestyle habits like?
- Do they keep a good schedule and routine?
- Do they drink enough water?
- Do they eat quality food?
- Are they getting quality sleep?

Is home maintenance becoming an issue?
- Are all the lights working in the house?
- Do they have rugs that need to be taped down?
- Are there carpeted areas that have lifted it up?
- Do they need help sorting through newspapers that have piled up?
- Do they have anything that needs to be moved that is too heavy to do?

How to Prevent Another Fall

If they fell outside:
- Check the vestibular system for balance issues
- Check the visual system to check depth perception and the ability to adjust to bright sunlight
- Were they using a device?
- Should they be considering using a device?
- Are their shoes fitting properly?

If exercise is the problem:
- Can they find a buddy to exercise with every day?
- Are there classes at their local senior center?
- Are they tech-savvy and could handle YouTube exercises?

If they fell in the shower:
- Would they be open to having grab bars installed?

- Would they consider it if they were hidden in place? There are lots of beautiful ones these days that improve the market value of a home.
- Would it be helpful to have a private caregiver come three days a week to supervise showers?
- Is there a place for them to sit down if they're dizzy or feeling low in blood sugar?

If they tripped on the way to the bathroom:
- Would they consider hardwiring in motion detector lights?
- Could they benefit from lights that come on automatically underneath the bed?
- Could they consider a shoe rack so shoes aren't left in the middle of the room and become a trip hazard?
- Do they need some help decluttering or prioritizing?
- Could a professional organizer be the catalyst to finally sort through 50 years of memories in boxes that are narrowing the hallway?

Falling Once Increases the Chances of Falling Again

It's so important to be proactive and prevent a second fall. Studies show that once you've had a fall, the chances of having another one are extremely likely in the following 30 days.

The biggest concern is that after a second fall, someone may develop a fear of falling, which then promotes a vicious cycle of even more falls. So, while there's nothing to panic about right now, it is important not to push it to the side either.

Ask the right questions so you can get on the right path.

Appendix B: Financial Help Resources

Is There Financial Help for Home Modifications?

Financial assistance for home modifications is available from many government and nonprofit organizations. Be sure to research your eligibility and look online for the latest information for assistance from all available sources, including but not limited to the following examples:

Federal Programs

- **Medicare Part B** will pay for a home safety assessment or evaluation, provided it is medically necessary and ordered by your primary care provider. Medicare will not cover the cost of home modification.
- The U.S. Department of Agriculture provides **Rural Housing Repair Loans and Grants** to rural homeowners with very low income. Grants up to $7,500 are available to homeowners age 62 and older. Loans, which don't have an age requirement, are available up to $20,000 and are repaid monthly over 20 years at an interest rate of one percent.
- The **Veterans Health Administration Home Improvements and Structural Alterations** grant provides funds for medically necessary home improvements, including accessibility updates to home entrances and bathrooms. The lifetime benefit is $6,800 for eligible veterans with a service-connected disability rated at 50 percent or more, or $2,000 lifetime benefit for eligible veterans with non-service-connected disabilities who receive health care from the VA.

Age in Place or Find a New Space

State and Local Programs

- Most states offer **Medicaid programs** that cover home modifications to enable older adults and/or disabled individuals to remain living at home. These will vary by diagnosis and state.
- The **U.S. Department of Housing and Urban Development** assists experienced nonprofit organizations, state and local governments, and public housing authorities in undertaking comprehensive programs that make safety and functional home modifications and limited repairs to meet the needs of low-income older adult homeowners. These efforts include the Older Adult Home Modification Program (OAHMP) and the Community Development Block Grant (CDBG) Program.
- Other **local nonprofits or faith communities** can also be a support.
  The **Eldercare Locator** is a public service of the U.S. Administration on Aging that connects caregivers to local services and resources for older adults.

Other Finance Options

- **Section 203(k) Rehab Mortgage Insurance** enables homebuyers and homeowners to finance both the purchase (or refinancing) of a house and the cost of its rehabilitation through a single mortgage or to finance the rehabilitation of their existing home.
- **Reverse mortgages** are a special type of loan that allows you to borrow against the equity that you've built up in your home. You must be at least age 62 to qualify. (Always consult your financial/tax advisor or lawyer for advice regarding your personal situation.)

Appendix C: Clinician Resources

PEO Model: How Do They Work Together?

PERSON: It Starts With You

How have you changed compared to what you used to do 10 years ago? As we age, our strength, balance, energy, and even memory can shift. In the PEO model, "Person" includes your current health, your medical diagnoses, but also your motivations, your routines, and your goals.

ENVIRONMENT: Your Space Must Work With You

Now imagine doing your daily routines, but with a walker. Or with arthritis in your hands. Or after a hospital stay. Most homes aren't built to flex with your changing needs. That's why environments matter so much. When your space isn't supporting you, it silently works against you.

OCCUPATION: What Makes Life Worth Living

These are your daily activities and roles: caring for a pet, cooking your favorite dish, bathing independently, gardening, and going to the book club. These tasks form the rhythm of your day—and they're exactly what we want to preserve. When those three areas are aligned, life flows. When they're out of sync, even simple tasks can feel impossible. The mission is to bring them back into harmony. So, how well you can do your job (occupational performance) is determined by how aligned the Person, Environment, and Occupation are.

How Evolving Homes® Aging in Place Model Connects to the PEO Model

Let's now tie it all together:
- **Person**: If you're weaker than you used to be, home modifications and fitness can bridge that gap.
- **Environment**: Smart tech and better layouts reduce risk.
- **Occupation**: Routines supported by coaching and design allow you to keep doing what matters most.

When we adjust just one piece of the puzzle, it helps—but when we adjust *all three*, life changes.

How to Use the PEO Model to Identify Solutions

The PEO model is dynamic, just like life. And when life starts to feel harder than it should, it's a good idea to pause and ask:
- Can I change something about *the person*? (Do I need rest, strength, support, connection?)
- Can I change something about *the environment*? (Could this space be safer, quieter, more efficient?)
- Can I adapt *the task*? (Is there a simpler, easier, more joyful way to do this?)

When even one of those three starts to shift, the others are affected. That's why creating a better fit between them is the secret to bringing all three domains back into harmony with each other.

To see how this looks in real life, I'd like you to meet a super-vibrant 92-year-old client who has lived alone for many years and is fiercely independent. Her loyal dog was 10 years old and could only eat canned food because he had lost many of his teeth. The brand that was recommended by her vet required a manual can opener, which initially was not a problem. However, after a few weeks, her hands started to feel weak and painful. Some days, she just couldn't puncture the top of the

Appendix C | Clinician Resources

can to get it started, and that forced her to ask a neighbor for help. Her occupational performance as a pet owner was suffering.

Step One: Investigate the Person
The Person is in pain, so that's the first priority—get the pain under control by addressing the inflammation with heat and ice and adding gentle range-of-motion exercises. I suggested using resting splints at night to reduce strain, but the answer was "I'll never remember to put those on." That self-awareness saved us from wasting time (and money) on solutions that wouldn't stick.

Step Two: Investigate the Environment
Once her pain was more manageable, we worked on positioning in the Environment. Could she open the cans while sitting at the table instead of standing at the counter? Could we stabilize her arms and the can for better leverage? Little tweaks helped, but not enough for the complete independence she was after.

Step Three: Investigate The Task
So, it was time to break down the Task and ask, "How could we change the task to improve performance?" Our short list of options was as follows:
1. Buy an electric can opener.
2. Ask the vet if a different, easier-to-open dog food was available.
3. Ask the neighbor to pre-open a week's worth of cans and store the food in easy-to-open containers.

So, despite her reluctance to rely on others, she ended up going with option three. Why is that?

Option one was rejected because she hates changing batteries. "Too much work," she said. "And what if I'm rushing to leave the house and the thing dies on me? No thanks." Option two was a non-negotiable. Her dog was getting the best food money could buy—period.

Age in Place or Find a New Space

In the end, option three turned out to be better than expected because she found a friendship that bloomed into regular Sunday night dinners with that neighbor, which included leftovers for her and prepped dog food for her pup, stored in a container she could open by herself ☺

Here's the thing: It can be easy to assume joint pain can only be addressed with traditional rehab methods. But in my experience, I have found that the most enduring solutions are the ones that embrace our individuality and align closely with our personal preferences. It may not seem like a big deal to you to change batteries, but to her, it was a deal-breaker.

As a client-centered clinician, my job is to continue looking for alternatives until she is satisfied with her functional level. I do this by systematically exploring the three key areas that influence occupational performance, using the PEO model as a guide to spark ideas. I encourage clients and their families to do the same when they're trying to find the right solution—for the right person, in the right situation, tackling the right task. Let's start by identifying the tasks that make up aging in place.

Appendix C | Clinician Resources

After a Fall: #OT Brain Investigation Questions

Demographics
- How old is the patient?
- Do they live alone?
- Do they have family nearby?
- How long have they lived in that location?
- What did they do for work?
- How long have they been retired?
- What kind of person are they? Active or normally sedentary?
- What do they enjoy doing for fun?

Injury Details
- What is the problem or concern? What injuries happened? What did they say happened? What do the family think happened?
- I like to draw out a timeline of events
- When that first event happened, was something different in the routine or situation? How long ago, or when, did the family start to see something change? Often this will be a year or more.
- Get lots of details about what the person says happened and what the theories are from the family about what might've happened
- Definitely want to know if something similar has happened before
- Were they supposed to be using equipment, and they weren't?
- Did they feel dizzy before they felt weak?

Medical Status
- What has been a common complaint?
- What is normal for them?
- Do you track blood pressure?
- Do you track water intake?
- Is there a past medical history of blood pressure problems? Dizziness? Blood sugar?

Age in Place or Find a New Space

- Do they have any difficulty with vision?
- Are they good water drinkers?
- Do they have a history of urinary tract infections?
- Do they have a history of feeling general weakness?
- Are they good with regular meals/ at maintaining good blood sugar?
- Do they get up to go to the bathroom at night? How many times?
- Do they turn on the lights to go to the bathroom?

Physical Clues
- Does the family notice if it's harder for them to get up and down from chairs? Do they have to help them?
- Is it harder to get in and out of the car?
- Walk with them and notice if you see dirt marks on the walls where they might be holding on/furniture, walking.

Environment
- Do they have any trouble getting in and out of bed?
- Can they get up and down from the toilet easily, or are they pulling on something?
- Is water on the floor frequently?
- Have they ever tripped on the steps? Usually, it's catching their toe on the end or misjudging the distance.

Normal Routines
- What do they normally do during the day?
- I'll usually ask them what time they wake up and get a timeline of literally what they're doing the whole day.

Appendix C | Clinician Resources

Current Situation
- What has changed since the fall? Usually, this is a change in behavior, like sitting more, using a walker, or avoiding social situations.

Solutions
- What solutions does the family think need to happen?
- What does the patient want?

Appendix D: Resources

AARP Care to Talk Cards

Online conversation cards to help start a meaningful discussion about healthcare, finances and future plans.

https://www.aarp.org/membership/benefits/caregiving/care-to-talk/

AARP Prepare to Care Guide

A caregiving planning guide for families to help guide conversations.

https://learn.aarp.org/prepare-to-care-guide

AARP Caregiving

Tips and support for family caregiving, from providing personal care, medical management and financial guidance to finding a healthy work-life balance. Free Caregiver Support Line: **1-877-333-5885.**

www.aarp.org/caregiving/

Area Agencies on Aging (AAA)

Local Area Agency on Aging (AAA) helps older adults remain in their homes by coordinating and offering services that vary by region. Meals-on-Wheels, homemaker assistance, and respite care services are some examples of services that may be offered. AAA are funded on a national level and refers to the Eldercare Locator to connect with services in your area.

Eldercare Locator

Search engine for local services for older adults and their families. **1-800-677-1116.**

https://eldercare.acl.gov/Public/index.aspx

Appendix D | Resources

National Alliance for Caregiving

A coalition of national organizations dedicated to improving quality of life for families and their care recipients through research, innovation, and advocacy.

www.caregiving.org

Center Independent Living—Temporary Loan Closet

The **Center for Independent Living (CIL)** is a pioneering organization founded in 1972 in Berkeley, California. It was the first independent living center in the United States, established by and for people with disabilities. CIL has been instrumental in the independent living movement, advocating for the rights, accommodations, and resources necessary for individuals with disabilities to live independently within their communities. Their services encompass advocacy, counseling, housing assistance, assistive technology, and more, all aimed at empowering individuals to lead self-sufficient lives
https://www.centerforindependentliving.org/

National Association of Professional Geriatric Care Managers

Aging Life Care™, also known as geriatric care management, is a holistic, client-centered approach to caring for older adults or others facing ongoing health challenges. Working with families, the expertise of Aging Life Care Professionals provides the answers at a time of uncertainty.

www.aginglifecare.org/

Age in Place or Find a New Space

Assisted Living by State Tool

The **Assisted Living by State** tool on AssistedLiving.org is a comprehensive resource designed to help older adults, caregivers, and families navigate the diverse landscape of assisted living across the United States. Recognizing that assisted living varies significantly from state to state—due to differences in care types, regulations, staffing requirements, and financial assistance—the Assisted Living Research Institute has compiled in-depth guides for each state. These guides provide valuable insights, including expert opinions and firsthand experiences from residents, to equip seniors with the knowledge they need to make informed decisions about assisted living in their specific state.

https://www.assistedliving.org/assisted-living-by-state/

Favorite Book Reference Resources:

1. *Can't We Talk About Something More Pleasant?* **by Roz Chast**
This graphic memoir by New Yorker cartoonist Roz Chast offers a candid and humorous exploration of her experience caring for her aging parents. Through a blend of cartoons, family photos, and narrative, Chast delves into the complexities of aging, family dynamics, and end-of-life care. The book has been praised for its honesty and was a finalist for the National Book Award.

2. *Build YOUR Space: How to Create an Accessible Home for You, Your Family, and Your Future,* **by Julie Sawchuk**
Julie Sawchuk, an accessibility strategist, shares her personal journey of designing and building an accessible home. The book provides practical advice on creating spaces that are safe, functional, and stylish, emphasizing the importance of planning for accessibility in home

Appendix D | Resources

design. Sawchuk combines her lived experience with expert insights to guide readers through the process.

3. *Universal Design Toolkit: Time-Saving Ideas, Resources, Solutions, and Guidance for Making Homes Accessible,* **by Rosemarie Rossetti** Rosemarie Rossetti offers a comprehensive guide to applying universal design principles in home construction and remodeling. Drawing from her experience building the Universal Design Living Laboratory, the book includes checklists, assessments, and practical tips to help readers create accessible and inclusive living spaces.

Low-Cost DME & Ramp Building Resources

- https://seniorsmobility.org/free-medical-equipment/near-me-national-programs/
- https://gotdme.org/
- Local church groups
- Local Council on Aging
- Lowe's Foundation
- Home Depot Foundation
- Goodwill thrift stores
- Temporary Loan Closet (Center of Independent Living)

Age in Place or Find a New Space

Practical Care & Daily Support

AARP Caregiving
Tips and support for family caregiving, from providing personal care, medical management, and financial guidance to finding a healthy work-life balance.
Free Caregiver Support Line: 877-333-5885
Nonprofit
www.aarp.org/caregiving/

Family Caregiver Alliance (FCA)
Practical caregiving tips, fact sheets, support groups, care navigation, and legal/financial tools.
Nonprofit
www.caregiver.org
https://www.linkedin.com/company/family-caregiver-alliance-fca/

Carers UK *(United Kingdom)*
Advice and community for unpaid carers, with guides on practical care, benefits, and working while caregiving.
Nonprofit/Charity
www.carersuk.org
https://www.linkedin.com/company/carers-uk/

Appendix D | Resources

Medical & Health Conditions

Alzheimer's Association
Education, 24/7 helpline, care planning, support groups, and research updates for dementia caregivers.
Helpline: 800-272-3900
Nonprofit
www.alz.org

Dementia Singapore *(Singapore)*
Caregiver training, helpline, therapy programs, and resource toolkits tailored to dementia care.
Nonprofit/IPC (Institution of a Public Character)
www.dementia.org.sg
LinkedIn

National Institute on Aging—Caregiving
Evidence-based advice on managing medications, preparing for medical visits, and understanding end-of-life issues.
U.S. Government/NIH Division (Nonprofit Equivalent)
www.nia.nih.gov/health/caregiving

Financial & Legal Guidance

Aging Life Care Association
Directory of certified aging life care professionals (geriatric care managers) who can help plan for health, legal, and financial needs.
Nonprofit Professional Association
www.aginglifecare.org

National Academy of Elder Law Attorneys (NAELA)
Find attorneys specializing in estate planning, long-term care, Medicaid, and disability rights.
Nonprofit Membership Organization
www.naela.org

End-of-Life Law Australia *(Australia)*
Free legal information, advance planning guides, and elder rights resources.
Nonprofit/Research Project Hosted by the University of Queensland
www.endoflifelaw.edu.au

Appendix D | Resources

Emotional Wellness & Respite

Caregiver Action Network
Peer support forums, stress management tools, care coordination tips, and weekly caregiver chats.
Nonprofit
www.caregiveraction.org

Circle of Care Podcast (Emory University)
Stories and practical tips for family caregivers caring for loved ones with chronic or serious illness.
Nonprofit (University-Backed)
Circle of Care Podcast

HelpGuide: Caregiver Stress & Burnout
Mental health guide for recognizing and managing emotional exhaustion in caregiving.
Nonprofit Mental Health Resource
www.helpguide.org/articles/stress/caregiving-stress-and-burnout.htm

Age in Place or Find a New Space

Technology & Tools

CareZone
A free app for managing meds, doctor notes, appointments, and a shareable care calendar.
For-Profit (acquired by Walmart Health)
www.carezone.com

Papa
A U.S.-based service connecting older adults and families with trained "Papa Pals" for companionship, tech help, and light assistance.
For-Profit/Startup
www.papa.com

TapestryCare (formerly, TapestryHealth)
Remote monitoring, virtual care services, and caregiver communication tools.
For-Profit Health Tech Company
www.tapestry.care

Appendix D | Resources

Home Modification & Aging in Place

Rebuilding Together
Provides free home repairs and modifications for low-income seniors across the U.S.
Nonprofit
www.rebuildingtogether.org

Habitat for Humanity—Aging in Place
Offers assessments and customized renovations to support independence at home.
Nonprofit/International
www.habitat.org/our-work/aging-in-place

Accessible Homes Australia (AHA) *(Australia)*
Promotes accessible housing design and offers housing support for people with disabilities and older adults.
Nonprofit/Disability Housing Advocate
www.accessiblehomes.org.au

Age in Place or Find a New Space

Home Assessment Platforms

AARP HomeFit
Free camera-based app that offers recommendations as you point to an object and provides a list of solutions.

Download app called *HomeFit AR*

Home for Life
A home safety assessment with Accessibility Ratings for consumers, enterprises, government agencies and payors. Contact for pricing.

www.homeforlifedesign.com

IncluzIT HOME
A free Aging and Home Safety planning tool design for public use.

www.incluzia.com

IncluzIT PRO
A customizable in depth home assessment platform for occupational therapists

www.Incluzia.com

Appendix D | Resources

Finding a Home Modification Occupational Therapist

U.S.-Based Resources

Home Modifications Occupational Therapy Alliance (HMOTA)
U.S.-based directory and community of OTs specializing in home safety and environmental interventions. Offers direct links to therapists offering assessments for aging in place.
Nonprofit Alliance (Membership-Based)
www.hmotalliance.org

AskSAMIE
Use the AskSAMIE platform to connect with qualified home modification occupational therapists in your area who specialize in aging in place.
https://www.asksamie.com/collections/featured-occupational-therapists

Capable Program (Johns Hopkins University)
While not a therapist directory, CAPABLE is a research-backed U.S. program that pairs low-income older adults with OTs and home repair professionals. Info is useful for caregivers seeking evidence-based models.
Nonprofit (University-Based Program)
www.nursing.jhu.edu/capable
https://www.linkedin.com/company/johns-hopkins-university-school-of-nursing/

American Occupational Therapy Association (AOTA)—Find an OT
Directory of licensed occupational therapists in the U.S., searchable by specialty (including home modifications, aging in place, and accessibility assessments). AOTA also offers resources on the role of OTs in fall prevention and safe aging.

Age in Place or Find a New Space

Nonprofit Professional Association
www.aota.org/Practice/Find-an-Occupational-Therapist
https://www.linkedin.com/company/american-occupational-therapy-association/

International Resources

Canadian Association of Occupational Therapists (CAOT)—Find an OT
National OT database searchable by province, service area (e.g., aging in place), and credentials. Includes French-language support and info on funding resources.
Nonprofit Professional Association
www.caot.ca
https://www.linkedin.com/company/caot/

Occupational Therapy Australia—Find an OT *(International – Australia)*
Nationwide OT directory including experts in home modifications and accessibility. Includes telehealth options for remote communities.
Nonprofit Professional Association
www.otaus.com.au/find-an-ot

World Federation of Occupational Therapists (WFOT)—Global Directory
Connects users with national OT associations worldwide, including countries in Asia, Europe, Africa, and Latin America. Each listing links to member organizations where caregivers can find qualified OTs.
Nonprofit International Federation
www.wfot.org/membership/member-organisations

Appendix D | Resources

Finding a Contractor for Home Modifications

U.S.-Based Resources

National Association of Home Builders (NAHB)—CAPS Directory
Directory of Certified Aging-in-Place Specialists (CAPS) trained in accessible design and modifications such as grab bars, ramps, stair lifts, and bathroom upgrades. Search by state and ZIP code.
For-Profit Trade Association
www.nahb.org/education-and-events/education/designations/certified-aging-in-place-specialist-caps

Rebuilding Together
Provides free home repairs and modifications for low-income seniors. Their affiliate network connects with skilled contractors and volunteers for safe aging-in-place upgrades.
Nonprofit
www.rebuildingtogether.org
https://www.linkedin.com/company/rebuilding-together/

Habitat for Humanity – Aging in Place Program
Offers home assessments and contractor services through its local chapters. Modifications focus on fall prevention, safety, and energy efficiency.
Nonprofit (International)
www.habitat.org/our-work/aging-in-place

HomeAdvisor—Senior and Disability Remodelers (U.S.)
Consumer-rated directory of licensed contractors for bathroom conversions, ramps, grab bars, and wider doorways. Filter by senior or disability remodel experience.
For-Profit / Part of Angi
www.homeadvisor.com

Age in Place or Find a New Space

Better Business Bureau (BBB)—Accredited Aging-in-Place Contractors
Use keyword searches like "aging-in-place" or "accessibility remodeling" to find rated and reviewed contractors. Ideal for vetting trustworthiness.
Nonprofit (Consumer Advocacy)
www.bbb.org

Canada-Specific Resources

March of Dimes Canada—Home & Vehicle Modification Program
Although this is a funding resource, they maintain a vetted list of contractors and suppliers who can implement safety renovations. Primarily serves Ontario, but guidance is transferable nationwide.
Nonprofit/Charity
www.marchofdimes.ca/en-ca/programs/hvmp
https://www.linkedin.com/company/march-of-dimes-canada/

Canadian Home Builders' Association (CHBA)—RenoMark Program
Certified renovator search tool, with members who follow aging-in-place and accessibility guidelines.
Nonprofit Trade Association
www.renomark.ca

International Options

Accessible Housing Australia—Contractor Guide
Educational resource for both homeowners and builders on how to create accessible and universally designed homes. Offers contractor references and project examples.
Nonprofit
www.accessiblehousing.org.au

Appendix D | Resources

UK Home Improvement Agencies (Found via Foundations UK)
A network of local nonprofit organizations across England that help older adults and disabled people find trusted contractors for home modifications.
Nonprofit Umbrella Organization
www.foundations.uk.com

Independent Living Centre Network (ILC Australia)
ILCs provide referrals to occupational therapists and home mod specialists, including contractors who are disability modification-certified.
Nonprofit Network
www.ilcaustralia.org.au

Finding Durable Medical Equipment

U.S.-Based Resources

AskSAMIE – OT built e-commerce platform
AskSAMIE makes it easy to find and compare home medical equipment that suits your needs, with guidance from therapists who understand accessibility.
https://www.asksamie.com/

Medicare.gov—DME Directory
Official site to find Medicare-approved suppliers for walkers, wheelchairs, oxygen tanks, hospital beds, and more. Also explains coverage and how to qualify.
Government/Nonprofit Equivalent
www.medicare.gov/coverage/durable-medical-equipment-dme-coverage

National Assistive Technology Act Technical Assistance and Training Center (AT3 Center)
State-by-state directory of programs offering free or low-cost assistive devices, equipment loans, and evaluations.
Federally Funded Nonprofit
www.at3center.net

Goodwill Home Medical Equipment (New Jersey/Philadelphia area)
Offers donated, refurbished medical equipment like scooters, hospital beds, and lift chairs at low cost.
Nonprofit
www.goodwillhomemedical.org

AbleData Archive (via National Rehabilitation Information Center)
Though no longer updated, its archived resources offer listings of suppliers for over 40,000 assistive technology products.

Appendix D | Resources

Formerly Government/Now Archived Resource
www.naric.com/?q=en/abledatadirectory

Numotion
National provider of power wheelchairs, mobility devices, ramps, and home access solutions. Works with insurance.
For-Profit (Largest U.S. DME Supplier)
www.numotion.com

Canada-Based Resources

Easter Seals Canada—Assistive Devices Programs
Provides funding assistance and helps locate affordable DME for children, youth, and adults with disabilities.
Nonprofit/Charity
www.easterseals.ca
https://www.linkedin.com/company/easter-seals-canada/

Canadian Red Cross Health Equipment Loan Program (HELP)
Offers short-term loans of walkers, bath chairs, canes, and crutches across most provinces.
Nonprofit/Charity
www.redcross.ca/in-your-community/health-equipment-loan-program

Ontario Assistive Devices Program (ADP)
Government program offering financial support for up to 75% of DME costs. Available to residents with long-term physical disabilities.
Government Program/Nonprofit Equivalent
www.ontario.ca/page/assistive-devices-program

International & Global Options

Independent Living Centres Australia (ILC)
Provides information, trials, and referrals for thousands of assistive

Age in Place or Find a New Space

technology and DME products. Includes an online "AT Database."
Nonprofit National Network
www.ilcaustralia.org.au

Motability (UK)
Offers adapted mobility vehicles and equipment through grants or rentals for people with disabilities.
Nonprofit/Charity
www.motability.org.uk

AGE Platform Europe – Assistive Technology Database
Advocacy group that links older adults to EU-wide assistive technology and accessible living services.
Nonprofit Network
www.age-platform.eu

WHO Assistive Technology Resources (Global)
Provides international guidance, standards, and directories on assistive products across low- and middle-income countries.
Public/NGO
www.who.int/health-topics/assistive-technology

Appendix D | Resources

Healthy Habits & Fitness Programs for Aging Adults

U.S.-Based Resources

National Institute on Aging—Exercise & Physical Activity Guide
Offers free evidence-based guides on strength, balance, flexibility, and endurance exercises for older adults. Includes printable workout plans and videos.
Government/Nonprofit Equivalent
www.nia.nih.gov/health/exercise-physical-activity

Go4Life® by NIA
Specialized workout program for older adults, including a fitness tracker, daily goals, and videos for every ability level.
Government Program (Under NIH)
www.go4life.nia.nih.gov

SilverSneakers
Fitness and wellness program available through many Medicare Advantage plans. Offers online and in-person classes including yoga, strength, walking groups, and fall prevention.
For-Profit/Insurance-Affiliated Program
www.silversneakers.com

YMCA Active Older Adults Programs
Local YMCAs offer fitness classes, social activities, and chronic disease management programs like "Enhance®Fitness" and "Moving for Better Balance."
Nonprofit
www.ymca.net/health/active-older-adults

Age in Place or Find a New Space

The Whole Person: Healthy Aging Toolkit
Self-care workbook and wellness planning tool developed for caregivers and older adults to improve nutrition, exercise, sleep, and routines.
Nonprofit (Created by Community-Based Health Orgs)
www.agingwithdignity.org/whole-person-wellness

Canada-Based Resources

Canadian Centre for Activity and Aging (CCAA)
National leader in older adult fitness education. Offers training for caregivers and instructors, and home-based exercise DVDs and printable plans.
Nonprofit (Part of Western University)
www.uwo.ca/ccaa

ParticipACTION—Stay Active at Any Age
Provides daily activity suggestions, workout videos, and "How to Start Moving More" guides tailored to older Canadians.
Nonprofit
www.participaction.com

Active Aging Canada
Delivers community-based programs and research-based fitness tips for seniors, plus fitness and cognitive health challenges.
Nonprofit/Charity
www.activeagingcanada.ca

Healthy Aging Core Canada—Physical Activity Resource Hub
Resource clearinghouse for community health workers and caregivers promoting active aging.
Nonprofit/Public Health Collaborative
www.healthyagingcore.ca

Appendix D | Resources

International Resources

Age UK—Fitness & Exercise at Home
Offers home fitness videos, walking challenges, and mobility guides for older adults.
Nonprofit/Charity
www.ageuk.org.uk/information-advice/health-wellbeing/exercise

WHO—Guidelines on Physical Activity for Older Adults
Provides global evidence-based recommendations for weekly movement, strength training, and activity modifications for seniors and those with chronic conditions.
International Public Health Organization
www.who.int/publications/i/item/9789240015128

Better Health (Australia)
Offers simple, accessible fitness routines, healthy eating plans, and daily habit-building tips for older adults.
Government/Public Health Resource
www.betterhealth.vic.gov.au

Move It or Lose It (UK)
Fun and easy home exercise program developed with physiotherapists. Offers DVDs, virtual classes, and chair-based fitness routines for all mobility levels.
Social Enterprise
www.moveitorloseit.co.uk

Age in Place or Find a New Space

Financial Assistance for Caregiving

U.S.-Based Resources

National Council on Aging (NCOA)—BenefitsCheckUp®
A free tool to find local, state, and federal programs that help pay for caregiving, medication, food, utilities, and more.
Nonprofit
www.benefitscheckup.org
https://www.linkedin.com/company/national-council-on-aging/

Medicaid Home and Community-Based Services (HCBS) Waivers
State-specific waivers may pay family caregivers, support home care, or fund respite and personal assistance services.
Government/Nonprofit Equivalent
www.medicaid.gov/medicaid/home-community-based-services

VA Aid & Attendance Benefit (Veterans Affairs)

Provides extra monthly income for veterans or surviving spouses who require help with daily living, including in-home care.
Government (Veterans Affairs)
www.va.gov/pension/aid-attendance-housebound

Family Caregiver Support Program (Administration for Community Living)
Federal funding distributed to states to provide caregiver education, counseling, respite, and limited financial help.
Government-Funded Program (ACL)
www.acl.gov/programs/support-caregivers

ARCH National Respite Network – Respite Funding Guide
State-by-state tool to find funding, vouchers, or grants for caregiver respite services.

Appendix D | Resources

Nonprofit
www.archrespite.org/respitelocator

Aid for Aging Parents: State-Paid Family Caregiver Programs
Overview of which U.S. states pay family caregivers directly, including eligibility and links to application portals.
Public Guide / Hosted by PayingForSeniorCare.com
www.payingforseniorcare.com/longtermcare/state-paid-family-caregiver

Canada-Based Resources

Canada Caregiver Credit (CCC)
Tax credit for those supporting a spouse, parent, or other dependent with a disability. Helps reduce taxable income.
Government Benefit
www.canada.ca/en/revenue-agency/services/tax/individuals/topics/about-your-tax-return/tax-return/completing-a-tax-return/deductions-credits-expenses/canada-caregiver-amount.html

Ontario's Family-Managed Home Care Program
Allows families to hire and pay caregivers directly (including family members) using funds managed through their local Home and Community Care Support Services.
Government Program
www.health.gov.on.ca/en/pro/programs/family_managed_care

March of Dimes Canada—Assistive Devices and Caregiver Support Programs
Provides grants and funding navigation for caregivers of individuals with disabilities.
Nonprofit/Charity
www.marchofdimes.ca

Employment Insurance (EI)—Caregiving Benefits
Canadian caregivers can apply for temporary income support (up to 35 weeks) to care for seriously ill family members.
Government Benefit
www.canada.ca/en/services/benefits/ei/caregiving.html

International Resources

Carer's Allowance—United Kingdom
Weekly financial benefit for people providing 35+ hours of unpaid care per week to someone receiving disability benefits.
Government Welfare Program (UK)
www.gov.uk/carers-allowance

Carers Australia—Financial Help for Carers
Offers info on carer payments, supplements, and concession programs available through Centrelink.
Nonprofit National Advocacy Org
www.carersaustralia.com.au

National Disability Insurance Scheme (NDIS)—Australia
Provides funding to people with disabilities for support services, including caregiver pay or respite funding.
Government Program
www.ndis.gov.au

Caregivers Alliance Limited (Singapore)
Nonprofit hub that offers financial navigation resources and government scheme info for caregivers in Singapore.
Nonprofit
www.cal.org.sg
https://www.linkedin.com/company/caregivers-alliance-limited/

Appendix D | Resources

Emotional Support, Self-Care & Support Groups for Caregivers

U.S.-Based Resources

Family Caregiver Alliance (FCA)
Offers online and in-person caregiver support groups, emotional wellness guides, stress checklists, and counseling referrals.
Nonprofit
www.caregiver.org
https://www.linkedin.com/company/family-caregiver-alliance-fca/

Caregiver Action Network (CAN)
Provides peer support forums, self-care resources, and a "Caregiver Help Desk" to connect with trained care advisors.
Nonprofit
Caregiver Help Desk: 855-227-3640
www.caregiveraction.org

ARCH National Respite Network—Caregiver Respite Locator
Helps caregivers find programs that offer emotional relief and short-term breaks. Includes self-care planning guides.
Nonprofit
www.archrespite.org

The Mighty—Caregiver Community
A digital storytelling platform and peer-led support forum where caregivers share experiences and support one another.
Free Platform Social Good Company
www.themighty.com/topic/caregivers

National Alliance for Caregiving (NAC)
Offers research, advocacy, and resources like "Circle of Care: Self-Care

for Caregivers" and caregiver mental health tools.
Nonprofit
www.caregiving.org
https://www.linkedin.com/company/national-alliance-for-caregiving/

Canada-Based Resources

Ontario Caregiver Organization (OCO)
24/7 Caregiver Helpline, peer support groups, mindfulness classes, and toolkits like "Caregiving Strategies" and "Self-Care 101."
Nonprofit
Caregiver Helpline: 1-833-416-2273
www.ontariocaregiver.ca
https://www.linkedin.com/company/the-ontario-caregiver-organization/

Wellness Together Canada
Free mental health and wellness support for caregivers, including self-paced courses, counseling, and peer support.
Government-Funded
www.wellnesstogether.ca

Canadian Virtual Hospice—MyGrief.ca & Caregiver Support Hub
Free online grief and caregiving modules developed by clinicians, with sections on coping, resilience, and finding meaning.
Nonprofit
www.virtualhospice.ca

Caregivers Alberta – COMPASS for the Caregiver
In-person and online support groups and learning series focused on building caregiver resilience and managing stress.
Nonprofit/Charity
www.caregiversalberta.ca

Appendix D | Resources

International Resources

Carers UK—Forum & Self-Care Hub
Offers 24/7 caregiver forums, emotional support guides, and mental health resources specifically for family carers.
Nonprofit/Charity
www.carersuk.org/help-and-advice/get-support/carers-uk-forum

Embracing Carers (Global Initiative)
Brings together global caregiver resources from across Europe, Asia, and the Americas. Includes a "Caregiver Well-Being Index" and tools for emotional support.
Global Campaign by Merck KGaA – Social Good Partnership
www.embracingcarers.com

Carers Australia—Mental Health & Respite Services
Provides one-on-one counseling, peer support, and carer self-care planning guides.
Nonprofit/Advocacy Organization
www.carersaustralia.com.au

iSupport for Dementia (WHO Tool—Global)
A free online training program from the World Health Organization with a strong focus on emotional regulation, stress relief, and coping skills.
Government/Public Health Tool (WHO)
www.who.int/publications/i/item/9789241515863

Driving Assessment & Transportation Alternatives for Older Adults

U.S.-Based Resources

AARP Driver Safety—We Need to Talk Program
Provides an online guide and conversation planner to help families determine when it's time to stop driving. Includes risk signs and self-assessment tools.
Nonprofit
www.aarp.org/auto/driver-safety/we-need-to-talk

American Occupational Therapy Association (AOTA)—Driving Specialists Directory
Search tool to find Certified Driver Rehabilitation Specialists (CDRS) who can assess driving skills, cognitive ability, and recommend adaptive equipment or retirement from driving.
Nonprofit Professional Association
www.aota.org/practice/older-drivers

AAA Senior Driving
Offers free online driving self-assessments, interactive visual perception tests, and resources to plan for driving retirement.
For-Profit (Social Good Division of AAA)
www.seniordriving.aaa.com

Ride Health
Coordinates non-emergency medical transportation (NEMT) for older adults through healthcare providers. Often covered by Medicaid or Medicare Advantage.
For-Profit Tech Company
www.ridehealth.com

Appendix D | Resources

GoGoGrandparent
A concierge ride service for seniors that works without a smartphone. Offers Lyft/Uber rides via phone call, plus medication delivery.
For-Profit Senior Service
www.gogograndparent.com

Canada-Based Resources

Canadian Association of Occupational Therapists (CAOT)—Driving Assessment OTs
Helps caregivers find licensed OTs offering functional driving assessments and referrals to provincial licensing boards.
Nonprofit
www.caot.ca/site/pd/driverassessment

Parachute Canada—Older Driver Safety Resources
Offers online decision tools for families and seniors, focusing on when to stop driving and what options exist.
Nonprofit Injury Prevention Org
www.parachute.ca/en/injury-topic/older-driver-safety

Driving Miss Daisy Canada
Offers escorted transportation services for older adults, including wheelchair assistance and accompaniment into appointments.
For-Profit (Senior Transportation Franchise)
www.drivingmissdaisy.ca

Transit App (Canada-wide)
Real-time public transit info and route planning across Canadian cities—ideal for seniors transitioning off driving.
For-Profit App/City Partnered
www.transitapp.com

Age in Place or Find a New Space

International Resources

OT Australia—Driving Assessments for Seniors
Offers a directory of OTs certified in driving assessments and rehabilitation services across Australia.
Nonprofit Professional Body
www.otaus.com.au/find-an-ot

Age UK-Transportation and Driving Support
Guides on knowing when to stop driving, getting assessed, and using community transport options.
Nonprofit/Charity
www.ageuk.org.uk/information-advice/travel-hobbies/driving

WHO Global Network for Age-friendly Cities – Mobility Tools
Encourages local programs that offer safe and accessible transport for older adults, especially in developing countries.
Public/NGO Program
www.who.int/initiatives/age-friendly-environments

Appendix D | Resources

Digital Literacy for Older Adults & Caregivers

U.S.-Based Resources

Senior Planet from AARP
Offers free online and in-person tech classes for seniors, including how to use smartphones, Zoom, social media, and online health portals.
Nonprofit (Part of Older Adults Technology Services – OATS at AARP)
www.seniorplanet.org
https://www.linkedin.com/company/senior-planet/

GetSetUp
Online platform offering live classes taught by older adults for older adults—topics include tech skills, online safety, and navigating telehealth. Free through many states and Medicare plans.
For-Profit Social Enterprise
www.getsetup.org

Cyber-Seniors
Intergenerational tech mentoring program that pairs older adults with youth mentors for digital coaching. Offers live webinars, one-on-one help, and online safety training.
Nonprofit
www.cyberseniors.org
https://www.linkedin.com/company/cyber-seniors/

TechBoomers
Free tutorial library designed for older adults covering websites, apps, and online safety (e.g. how to use YouTube, Facebook, Zoom, and more).
Free Public Resource (Education Site – Ad-supported)
www.techboomers.com

Age in Place or Find a New Space

Canada-Based Resources

Connected Canadians
Delivers one-on-one digital literacy training for older adults across Canada, led by volunteers and tech mentors. Sessions are remote or in person.
Nonprofit
www.connectedcanadians.ca
https://www.linkedin.com/company/connected-canadians/

ABC Life Literacy – Digital Literacy Program
Offers easy-to-understand tutorials on using email, smartphones, and social media for older adults. Many materials available in multiple languages.
Nonprofit
www.abclifeliteracy.ca
https://www.linkedin.com/company/abc-life-literacy-canada/

International Resources

Digital Unite (UK)
Provides free printable guides and online tutorials designed for older people and caregivers. Topics include online safety, Zoom, email, and banking online.
Social Enterprise / Nonprofit-Style
www.digitalunite.com

Be Connected (Australia)
A government-funded digital literacy platform with interactive lessons, courses, and community support to help older Australians stay connected and safe online.
Public Initiative by Good Things Foundation + Australian Govt.

Appendix D | Resources

www.beconnected.esafety.gov.au
https://www.linkedin.com/company/good-things-foundation/

Generations Working Together—Digital Inclusion Toolkit (Scotland)
Promotes digital literacy by connecting older adults and younger volunteers through tech training and shared learning activities.
Nonprofit/Charity
www.generationsworkingtogether.org

Protecting Seniors from Online Scams & Financial Exploitation

U.S.-Based Resources

AARP Fraud Watch Network
Scam alerts, educational webinars, a scam-tracking map, and a free helpline to help protect older adults from fraud, including phishing, tech scams, and caregiver financial abuse.
Nonprofit
Helpline: 877-908-3360
www.aarp.org/money/scams-fraudhttps://www.linkedin.com/showcase/aarp-fraud-watch-network/

Consumer Financial Protection Bureau (CFPB)—Older Adults Financial Protection
Offers "Managing Someone Else's Money" guides, scam prevention tips, and caregiver protections around legal and financial authority.
Government Agency
www.consumerfinance.gov/older-americans

Federal Trade Commission (FTC)—Elder Fraud Resources
Provides scam alerts, complaint reporting tools, and educational materials on common senior-targeted fraud tactics like romance scams and fake tech support.
Government Agency
www.consumer.ftc.gov

National Center on Elder Abuse (NCEA)
Education and guidance on identifying and reporting elder financial exploitation and caregiver misconduct.
Government-Funded (Hosted by USC)
www.ncea.acl.gov

Appendix D | Resources

National Adult Protective Services Association (NAPSA)
Helps families report suspected financial abuse by caregivers or others. Includes a state-by-state abuse reporting directory.
Nonprofit
www.napsa-now.org

Canada-Based Resources

Canadian Anti-Fraud Centre (CAFC)
Tracks active scams in Canada and educates seniors on phishing, grandparent scams, tech fraud, and identity theft. Accepts direct fraud reports.
Government/Public Safety Partnership
Report Line: 1-888-495-8501
www.antifraudcentre-centreantifraude.ca

Canadian Centre for Cyber Security—Seniors Online Safety Guide
Practical guidance on creating secure passwords, recognizing scams, and staying safe while banking and shopping online.
Government Cybersecurity Unit
www.cyber.gc.ca/en/guidance/seniors

Seniors Safety Line (Ontario)
24/7 confidential helpline for older adults facing fraud, coercion, or caregiver financial abuse. *Nonprofit – Assaulted Women's Helpline Program*
Helpline: 1-866-299-1011
www.awhl.org/seniors-safety-line

Public Guardian and Trustee (Province-Specific)
Investigates misuse of power of attorney and financial exploitation by professionals or family caregivers.
Government/Public Service
Example: www.trustee.bc.ca

Age in Place or Find a New Space

International Resources

Hourglass (UK) – Safer Aging and Financial Abuse Reporting
Offers support for those experiencing financial abuse by caregivers or scammers. Includes a confidential helpline and elder justice resources.
Nonprofit/Charity
Helpline: 0808 808 8141
www.wearehourglass.org

Be Connected (Australia)
Offers senior-friendly online safety classes, guides on scam awareness, and digital confidence-building to reduce fraud vulnerability.
Government Funded (with Good Things Foundation)
www.beconnected.esafety.gov.au

HelpAge International – Global Elder Protection Resources
Focuses on elder rights and protection from financial exploitation in low- and middle-income countries.
Nonprofit/NGO
www.helpage.org
https://www.linkedin.com/company/helpage-international/

World Health Organization – Global Elder Abuse Toolkit
Outlines risk factors and prevention strategies for financial abuse and online scams targeting older adults.
Public Health / NGO
www.who.int/news-room/fact-sheets/detail/elder-abuse

Appendix D | Resources

Disease-Specific Foundations & Support Organizations

Alzheimer's & Dementia

Alzheimer's Association (U.S.)
Support groups, a 24/7 helpline, care planning, and dementia education for caregivers.
Nonprofit
Helpline: 1-800-272-3900
www.alz.org
https://www.linkedin.com/company/alzheimer's-association/

Alzheimer's Society (UK)
Online caregiver courses, dementia advisors, and a dementia-friendly community guide.
Nonprofit/Charity
www.alzheimers.org.uk

Cancer

American Cancer Society
Offers caregiver resources, support hotlines, cancer treatment guides, and lodging help during treatment.
Nonprofit
Helpline: 1-800-227-2345
www.cancer.org

CancerCare
Provides counseling, support groups, and financial help for people living with cancer and their families.
Nonprofit
www.cancercare.org

Diabetes

American Diabetes Association (ADA)
Offers meal planning, medication management, foot care tips, and resources for caregivers of people with Type 1 and Type 2 diabetes.
Nonprofit
www.diabetes.org

Diabetes Canada
Programs and publications for managing diabetes at home, caregiver webinars, and prevention tips.
Nonprofit
www.diabetes.ca

Heart Disease

American Heart Association (AHA)
Resources on heart failure, blood pressure, cholesterol, stroke prevention, and caregiver education.
Nonprofit
www.heart.org

Heart & Stroke Foundation of Canada
Caregiver-specific support, rehab recovery tools, and healthy lifestyle programs.
Nonprofit
www.heartandstroke.ca

Lung Disease

American Lung Association (ALA)
Resources for COPD, asthma, lung cancer, and pulmonary rehab. Includes a Lung HelpLine for caregivers and patients.

Appendix D | Resources

Nonprofit
Lung HelpLine: 1-800-LUNGUSA (586-4872)
www.lung.org

Canadian Lung Association
Lung health information and patient resources for breathing disorders, with caregiver toolkits.
Nonprofit
www.lung.ca

Stroke

National Stroke Association (now part of AHA/ASA)
Information on post-stroke caregiving, speech and mobility rehab, and family education.
Nonprofit (via American Stroke Association)
www.stroke.org

Stroke Recovery Association of BC (Canada)
Resources for survivors and caregivers including group support and mobility programs.
Nonprofit
www.strokerecoverybc.ca

Parkinson's Disease

Parkinson's Foundation (U.S.)
Free Helpline, "Aware in Care" hospital kit, caregiver guides, and local support networks. *Nonprofit*
Helpline: 1-800-4PD-INFO
www.parkinson.org

Davis Phinney Foundation

Age in Place or Find a New Space

Focuses on helping people with Parkinson's live well today. Offers practical resources like exercise videos, caregiver guides, live webinars, and the Every Victory Counts® manual, which provides proactive, daily strategies for living with Parkinson's.
Nonprofit
www.davisphinneyfoundation.org

American Parkinson Disease Association (APDA)

Provides a wide range of resources including a national helpline, educational materials, caregiver support, local chapters, exercise classes, and community events. Also offers a free "Spotlight on Parkinson's Disease" webinar series.
Nonprofit
Helpline: 1-800-223-2732
www.apdaparkinson.org

Michael J. Fox Foundation for Parkinson's Research (MJFF)

Focused on funding research to find a cure and offering practical resources for living with Parkinson's. Provides a free Parkinson's guide, webinar series, caregiver content, and a clinical trial matching tool.
Nonprofit
www.michaeljfox.org

Parkinson Canada
Caregiver resources, webinars, and a toll-free info line to support disease management.
Nonprofit
www.parkinson.ca

Appendix D | Resources

Arthritis

Arthritis Foundation (U.S.)
Exercise programs, daily living tips, and pain management tools for caregivers and individuals.
Nonprofit
www.arthritis.org

Arthritis Society Canada
Self-management programs, pain tracking tools, and caregiving support services. *Nonprofit/Charity*
www.arthritis.ca

ALS (Lou Gehrig's Disease)

ALS Association (U.S.)
Provides caregiver guides, home safety tips, clinical trial access, and mobility planning.
Nonprofit
www.als.org

ALS Society of Canada
Caregiver resources, equipment loan programs, and support groups.
Nonprofit
www.als.ca

Multiple Sclerosis (MS)

National Multiple Sclerosis Society (U.S.)
Offers caregiving guides, mobility resources, mental health support, and community events.
Nonprofit
www.nationalmssociety.org

Age in Place or Find a New Space

MS Society of Canada
Support services, education events, and caregiver advocacy resources.
Nonprofit
www.mssociety.ca

Acknowledgements

To my wonderful husband, Justin, and my amazing kids, Dane and Luxe, thank you for getting in the boat and taking this journey with me. We left the comfort of the mainland so I could search for a place where I could truly make an impact. I'm forever grateful for your trust in me.

To my business besties, Sydney and Dawn—our 20-year age gap and diverse focus areas in the home modification world have made our friendship incredibly rich (and full of late-night laughs). I will always be grateful for KBIS 2023 and CTJWD. Where would I be without you guys??!

To my parents, Ping and Chin, thank you for raising my sisters, Marylyn and Ruth, and me to understand and respect money without shame or stigma. Because of you, my children are growing up in an environment where financial literacy is not only normalized but also encouraged. Mom, you taught us that money is not the goal—it's simply a tool. Thank you.

To my in-laws—Molly, Ted, and Shelley—Thank you for your wisdom during my deep dives into entrepreneurship. Your steady presence has meant the world to me.

To my brilliant, problem-solving bestie, Mary Ellen—I laugh when our kids say that we sound exactly like each other. I am utterly grateful to have you in my life. Thank you for 15 years of friendship and brainstorming power walks. I honestly don't know where I'd be without you.

To my mentors, Dr. Jim and Kathy M.—I really have no way to express the magnitude of my gratefulness for the intense support you have both shown me over the last 18 years. Thank you for catching me when I stumble and helping me see that everything is about mindset.

To my IIX CARE family—Edward, Alexandros, HaeJin, Marco, Rama, Ted, and Carolynne—I'm so grateful to work with such an incredible team so driven by purpose. It's an honor for me to build meaningful, impactful initiatives with you all every single day.

Age in Place or Find a New Space

To my favorite adventurer-at-heart, Debbie H.—I'm not kidding when I say that everything in my life can somehow be traced back to you. Our friendship holds a special place in my heart, and I love nothing more than spending time hatching big plans with you. You are the best.

To Melanie L., thank you for being the PT to my OT. Who knew two student-athletes from McGill would turn into partners 25 years later? My business is better because of your unwavering support.

To Laura C-P., the world of OTs in technology is small and I'm so grateful for your support. Thank you for reading drafts and offering such valuable feedback.

To the late Mark Gray + Sherri S.—working on "No Place Like Home" grew my brain so much and introduced me to Monica S.+ Kim C, two of the kindest souls I've ever met. What a gift.

To Carolyn M—Thank you for always lifting others up with your ROCs: Resources, Opportunities, and Connections. I'm so grateful for your support and belief in me.

To Patti B — I'm indebted to Dr. Joe for introducing us. You are amazing and inspiring. I'm so grateful to know such a warm human being who truly cares. Thank you for all your cheers.

To Dr. Joe, founder of MIT AgeLab—thank you for inviting me to speak at the 2023 PLAN Forum. That event sparked my interest in the financial side of aging, which started this book.

To my favorite people at TRI—Kate, Rune, Bisi, Leticia, Rishabh, Eric, Reko and my UK colleagues, Will K, Matt P. It's been an honor to collaborate with such brilliant minds. I'll never forget watching Baymax in action with my kids and thinking – wow, amazing that this is my life!

To Liz B. and Bob S. at AARP—Thank you for the opportunity to join *"Conversations for the Future: Finances, Health, and Housing"* with Amy G. and Amanda S. It was an honor.

To my ReThinking Aging Club—Debbie, Linda, Ray, Ellen, Elizabeth—I love all the fun we have attending conferences together. I hope that never ends ☺

Acknowledgments

To the Carter Japan Market Research Group & friends—Dom, Debbie, Adam, Asako, and our InAge gang Ginger G., Clare C., Bailey P., Dan R., Idit R.—Thank you for the adventure and the opportunities, the delicious food, and for warmly welcoming me to Japan.

To my WBO sisters—Laurie L. and Diane F., whose editorial expertise helped shape this book—I'm grateful for your clarity and guidance.

To Sam and Mary F., and Paul and Linda T., thank you for taking the wild ride with me to film No Place Like Home. I can't thank you enough for trusting me to tell your stories.

To my fellow McGill OTs and PTs—Jane H, Marco F, May L, Hyman G, Nina T, I'm grateful for the enduring friendships and our support of each other as we enter our 50s.

To my 514 girls—Claire R, Lisa P, Erika D, Heather B, so glad for your friendship after so many decades.

To my Korea friends — Carole C, Heather G, Lindsay M, Renee S. What a wild, wild west adventure we had together. So many memories, so much fun and laughter!

Finally, to my clients, readers, and fellow OTs—this book exists because of you:

OTs make sense out of chaos and build bridges between disciplines, values, and people. Our life experiences, empathy, and creativity are central to the healing process, and that's what makes occupational therapy so powerful and so necessary.

Even when misunderstood by the public ("Thanks, but I don't need OT—I'm retired"), we keep showing up. I'm here to say to you all: Be *proud* that we don't fit neatly in the Medicare box. We are the secret sauce. We are the ones who ask, "What matters most to you?"…And then figure out how to make that happen, no matter what it takes! #otbrain #professionalproblemsolve

About the Author

Carol Chiang, OTR/L, CAPS, ECHM, CHAMP, globally recognized aging-in-place expert, occupational therapist, Parkinson's advocate, and host of a MedBridge podcast called *Innovative Aging*.

With 27 years of clinical experience and a reputation for blending practicality with compassion, Carol focuses on person-centered design that empowers individuals and supports caregivers. A graduate of McGill University in Canada, she began her career in the U.S. at Brooks Rehab—one of the nation's premier inpatient rehabilitation facilities—before spending over a decade in home health, gaining a deep, firsthand understanding of the real-life challenges older adults and caregivers face in their homes.

As the founder of Evolving Homes®, Carol created Age in Place or Find a New Space®, a service that helps families confidently decide whether remodeling or relocating will better support their needs, values, and long-term quality of life. Her work is not just about grab bars—it's about understanding the person, their environment, their caregivers, and crafting solutions that preserve dignity, independence, and human connection.

An engaging speaker and educator, Carol is a frequent guest lecturer for occupational therapy programs and graduate students in architecture and design, where she emphasizes the importance of person-centered environments and interdisciplinary collaboration. She shares real-world insights that help students better understand the challenges and mindsets of the older adults they are designing for. Her goal is to combine clinical reasoning and design thinking to inspire the next generation of professionals. Carol's expertise is trusted by leading organizations such as MIT AgeLab, Toyota Research Institute, AARP, and UBS.

She has presented globally on topics ranging from smart home technology to the future of housing for aging populations and has led national webinars for the National Kitchen and Bath Association, AARP, and the Davis Phinney Foundation.

About the Author

In 2021, she filmed a pilot TV show, No Place Like Home, which explored luxury aging-in-place solutions and emerging technologies that support independence.

She was recently published in *Applied Sciences* for a peer-reviewed article on robotic caregiving: "Exploring Embodiment Form Factors of a Home-Helper Robot," which examines how robotic design can develop a trusting relationship and improve caregiver support in the home.

A McGill Sports Hall of Fame inductee and Olympic-caliber swimmer, Carol brings the same resilience, curiosity, and relentless drive to solve complex challenges to her work in healthcare innovation. She is a dynamic speaker known for reframing aging as a season of empowerment, innovation, and opportunity—not decline.

Endnotes

Chapter One

[i] AARP Press Release. "AARP Survey Shows 8 in 10 Older Adults Want to Age in Their Homes, While the Number and Needs of Households Headed by Older Adults Grow Dramatically." November 18, 2021. Accessed November 8, 2024.
https://www.press.aarp.org/2021-11-18-AARP-Survey-Shows-8-in-10-Older-Adults-Want-to-Age-in-Their-Homes-While-Number-and-Needs-of-Households-Headed-Older-Adults-Grow-Dramatically.

[ii] Harvard Health Letter. "Why We Should Exercise – and Why We Don't." August 26, 2019. Accessed November 14, 2024.
https://www.health.harvard.edu/newsletter_article/why-we-should-exercise-and-why-we-dont

[iii] Sussman, Tamara and Bianca Tétrault. "People Are More Afraid of a Dementia Diagnosis than of Death." Frontiers Dementia, Vol. 1 - 2022.
(https://doi.org/10.3389/frdem.2022.1043661.)
https://www.frontiersin.org/journals/dementia/articles/10.3389/frdem.2022.1043661/full
Accessed June 6, 2025.

[iv] Dunstan, D. W., Howard, B., Healy, G. N., & Owen, N. (2012). *Too much sitting: A health hazard.* Diabetes Research and Clinical Practice. Accessed June 6, 2025. 97(3), 368–376. https://doi.org/10.1016/j.diabres.2012.05.020.

Endnotes

ᵛ Genworth Cost of Care Survey Calculator. Accessed November 15, 2024. https://www.genworth.com/aging-and-you/finances/cost-of-care

Chapter Two

ᵛⁱⁱ Herlihy, Jim. "Honoring 16 Million+ Alzheimer's Caregivers." AARP. Accessed June 6, 2025. https://states.aarp.org/colorado/honoring-16-million-alzheimers-caregivers

ᵛⁱⁱⁱ Law, M., Cooper, B., Strong, S., Stewart, D., Rigby, P., & Letts, L. (1996). Accessed June 1, 2025 The Person-Environment-Occupation Model: A Transactive Approach to Occupational Performance. Canadian Journal of Occupational Therapy, 63(1), 9–23. https://doi.org/10.1177/000841749606300103

Chapter Four

ⁱˣ Reggev, Kate. Architectural Digest. "The ADA-Compliant Design Is paving the Way for Accessible Design. August 4, 2020. Accessed March 14, 2025. https://doh.colorado.gov/home-modification-tax-credit

ⁱˣ AARP Press Release. "AARP Survey Shows 8 in 10 Older Adults Want to Age in Their Homes, While the Number and Needs of Households Headed by Older Adults Grow Dramatically." November 18, 2021. Accessed November 8, 2024. https://www.press.aarp.org/2021-11-18-AARP-Survey-Shows-8-in-10-Older-Adults-Want-to-Age-in-Their-Homes-While-Number-and-Needs-of-Households-Headed-Older-Adults-Grow-Dramatically.

Chapter Six

ˣ Atsushi Yamamoto et al., "Prevalence and Risk Factors of a Rotator Cuff Tear in the General Population," Accessed May 3, 2025. *Journal of Shoulder and Elbow Surgery* 19, no. 1 (2010): 116–120, https://doi.org/10.1016/j.jse.2009.04.006.

ˣⁱ Cooper Design Builders, "How Much Will Your Portland Home Remodel Increase the Sale Price?" *Cooper Design Builders Blog*, accessed June 14, 2025, https://blog.cooperdesignbuilders.com/portland-home-remodel-increase-sale-price-home-value

xii Sal Alfano, "Bath Remodel—Universal Design," *Journal of Light Construction*, January 2024, Accessed May 3, 2025. https://www.jlconline.com/cost-vs-value/bath-remodel-universal-design?y=2024

xiii Ulrich, R. S. (1984). *View through a window may influence recovery from surgery*. **Science**, 224(4647), 420–421. https://doi.org/10.1126/science.6143402. Accessed 6/10/2025

xiv Centers for Disease Control and Prevention. "Data & Research: Older Adult Falls." Last modified June 20, 2024. Accessed June 10, 2025 https://www.cdc.gov/falls/data-research/index.html.

Chapter Eight

xv Dr. Peter Attia, "Why Mainstream Medicine Struggles to Prevent Chronic Disease—and What You Can Do About It," *GQ*, March 29, 2023. Accessed June 2,2025

xvi American Medical Association. "Living with Chronic Pain, Lifespan vs Healthspan, and Updated Dietary Guideline Recommendations." *AMA Update*, December 18, 2024. Accessed June 2, 2025

xvii Garmany, Armin, Satsuki Yamada, and Andre Terzic. 2021. Accessed June 2, 2025 "Longevity Leap: Mind the Healthspan Gap." *npj Regenerative Medicine* 6 (1): 57. https://doi.org/10.1038/s41536-021-00169-5.

xviii Springer, Jo-Ann, et al. "Prevalence and Prevention of Urinary Tract Infections Among Older Adults: A Systematic Review." *Journal of Aging & Social Policy*, vol. 36, no. 1, 2024. Accessed June 13, 2025 https://link.springer.com/article/10.1007/s12126-024-09569-6.

xix Office of Disease Prevention and Health Promotion. "Reduce the Rate of Hospital Admissions for Urinary Tract Infections Among Older Adults — OA-07." *Healthy People 2030*, U.S. Department of Health and Human Services. Accessed June 25, 2025. https://odphp.health.gov/healthypeople/objectives-and-data/browse-objectives/infectious-disease/reduce-rate-hospital-admissions-urinary-tract-infections-among-older-adults-oa-07.

xx Foxman, Betsy, Kaleb D. Yohannes, Peter M. DeRosa, and Amy E. Krambeck. "Evaluation of Recurrent Urinary Tract Infection Frequency Among Female Patients in the US." *JAMA Internal Medicine* 184, no. 6 (2024): 615–622. Accessed June 25, 2025 https://jamanetwork.com/journals/jamainternalmedicine/fullarticle/2819818

www.ingramcontent.com/pod-product-compliance
Lightning Source LLC
LaVergne TN
LVHW091702070526
838199LV00050B/2260